H. Toshima · Y. Koga · H. Blackburn (Editors)
A. Keys (Honorary Editor)

Lessons for Science
from
the Seven Countries Study

A 35-Year Collaborative Experience
in Cardiovascular Disease Epidemiology

With 49 Figures

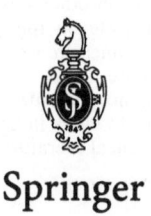

Springer

Honorary Editor:
ANCEL KEYS, M.D.
Emeritus Professor, Division of Epidemiology, School of Public Health, University of
Minnesota, MN 55454, USA

Editors:
HIRONORI TOSHIMA, M.D.
Emeritus Professor, The Third Department of Medicine, The Institute of
Cardiovascular Diseases, Kurume University School of Medicine, Kurume, 830 Japan

YOSHINORI KOGA, M.D.
Associate Professor, The Third Department of Medicine, Kurume University School of
Medicine, Kurume, 830 Japan

HENRY BLACKBURN, M.D.
Mayo Professor of Public Health and Professor of Medicine, Division of Epidemiology,
School of Public Health, University of Minnesota, MN 55454, USA

Front cover: Stadium Gate 27 of the University of Minnesota, where the Seven
Countries Study began.

ISBN-13:978-4-431-68271-4   e-ISBN-13:978-4-431 68269 1
DOI: 10.1007/978-4-431-68269-1

© Springer-Verlag Tokyo 1994
Softcover reprint of the hardcover 1st edition 1994

Typesetting: Best-set Typesetter Ltd., Hong Kong

Preface

The Seven Countries Study has made central contributions to the understanding of the socio-cultural influences on population rates of cardiovascular diseases (CVD). It has pointed the way to preventive strategies for whole populations. The Study is unique as a long-term investigation, now in its 35th year.

This pioneering work arose in part from a meeting between Professors Ancel Keys and Noboru Kimura to discuss differences observed in clinical manifestations and pathology of coronary disease in the U.S. and Japan. Professor Keys started explorations of the importance in these differences of dietary fat and serum cholesterol when he visited Japan in 1954, and thereafter initiated the Seven Countries Study to test these hypotheses.

In the Japanese cohorts of the Study, it became evident from the outset that coronary artery disease was extremely rare, but its incidence has since increased along with dramatic lifestyle changes from traditional Japanese to western styles. The Japanese experience contrasts with a reduction in coronary artery disease in many western countries along with establishment of major preventive efforts in risk factor reduction and cardiac care.

This International Symposium: "Lessons for Science from the Seven Countries Study" was proposed to celebrate the 35th anniversary of the Seven Countries Study as well as the 90th birthday of Professor Keys. It also highlighted concerns over the risk of a future coronary disease epidemic in Japan. The International Symposium was held successfully on October 30, 1993 in Fukuoka, Japan. It was attended by 17 of the principal investigators or their successors, and many visiting colleagues from several countries. In addition to reviews and progress reports from the Seven Countries Study, special lectures were given by the invited speakers, Professor Frederick Epstein from Switzerland and Professor Jeremiah Stamler from the U.S. The only regret of the editors and participants was the absence from the meeting of the late Professor Noboru Kimura, pioneer in cardiovascular disease research and prevention.

This volume includes all presentations of the Symposium with discussion. The editors gratefully acknowledge the contributions of all authors.

H. Toshima, Y. Koga, and H. Blackburn

Contents

Part 4. Lessons from the Seven Countries Study

List of Contributors

Adachi, Hisashi
The Third Department of Medicine, Kurume University School of Medicine, 67 Asahimachi, Kurume, 830 Japan

Blackburn, Henry
Division of Epidemiology, School of Public Health, University of Minnesota, 1300 S. 2nd St., Suite 300, Minneapolis, MN 55454, USA

Bloemberg, Bennie P.M.
Division of Public Health Research, National Institute of Public Health and Environmental Protection, Antonie van Leeuwenhoeklaan 9, 3720 BA, Bilthoven, The Netherlands

Dontas, Anastasios S.
Athens Home for the Aged, 137 Kifissias, 115-24 Athens, Greece

Epstein, Frederick H.
Institute of Social and Preventive Medicine, University of Zürich, Klausstrasse 4, CH8008 Zürich, Switzerland

Feskens, Edith
National Institute of Public Health and Environmental Protection, Antonie van Leeuwenhoeklaan 9, 3720 BA, Bilthoven, The Netherlands

Fidanza, Adalberta Alberti
Istituto di Scienza dell'Alimentazione, Univesità degli Studi, 06100 Perugia, Italy

Fidanza, Flaminio
Istituto di Scienza dell'Alimentazione, Univesità degli Studi, 06100 Perugia, Italy

Giampaoli, Simona
Laboratory of Epidemiology and Biostatistics, Istituto Superiore di Sanità, Viale Regina Elena 299, 00161 Rome, Italy

Grujić, Miodrag Z.
Institute for Cardiovascular Diseases, University Clinical Center, Koste Todorovica 8, 11000 Belgrade, Yugoslavia

Hannan, Peter J.
Division of Epidemiology, School of Public Health, University of Minnesota, 1300 S. 2nd St., Suite 300, Minneapolis, MN 55454, USA

Hashimoto, Ryuichi
The Third Department of Medicine, Kurume University School of Medicine, 67 Asahimachi, Kurume, 830 Japan

Jacobs, Jr., David R.
Division of Epidemiology, School of Public Health, University of Minnesota, 1300 S. 2nd St., Suite 300, Minneapolis, MN 55454, USA

Karvonen, Martti
84060 Pioppi SA, Italy

Keys, Ancel
Division of Epidemiology, School of Public Health, University of Minnesota, 1300 S. 2nd St., Suite 300, Minneapolis, MN 55454, USA

Kivelä, Sirkka-Liisa
Department of Public Health Science and General Practice, University of Oulu, Aapistie 1, FIN-90220 Oulu, Finland

Kivinen, Paula
Department of Community Health and General Practice, University of Kuopio, P.O. Box 1627, Harjulantie 1 B, FIN-70211 Kuopio, Finland

Koga, Yoshinori
The Third Department of Medicine, Kurume University School of Medicine, 67 Asahimachi, Kurume, 830 Japan

Kromhout, Daan
Division of Public Health Research, National Institute of Public Health and Environmental Protection, Antonie van Leeuwenhoeklaan 9, 3720 BA, Bilthoven, The Netherlands

McGovern, Paul G.
Division of Epidemiology, School of Public Health, University of Minnesota,
1300 S. 2nd St., Suite 300, Minneapolis, MN 55454, USA

Menotti, Alessandro
Laboratory of Epidemiology and Biostatistics, Istituto Superiore di Sanità,
Viale Regina Elena 299, 00161 Rome, Italy

Nedeljković, Srecko I.
Institute for Cardiovascular Diseases, University Clinical Center, Koste
Todorovica 8, 11000 Belgrade, Yugoslavia

Nissinen, Aulikki
Department of Community Health and General Practice, University of Kuopio,
P.O. Box 1627, Harjulantie 1 B, FIN-70211 Kuopio, Finland

Ostojić, Miodrag Č.
Institute for Cardiovascular Diseases, University Clinical Center, Koste
Todorovica 8, 11000 Belgrade, Yugoslavia

Pekkanen, Juha
Department of Environmental Epidemiology, National Public Health Institute,
P.O. Box 95, 70071 Kuopio, Finland

Puska, Pekka
Department of Epidemiology and Health Promotion, National Public Health
Institute, SF-00510 Helsinki, Finland

Ripsin, Cynthia M.
Division of Epidemiology, School of Public Health, University of Minnesota,
1300 S. 2nd St., Suite 300, Minneapolis, MN 55454, USA

Seccareccia, Fulvia
Laboratory of Epidemiology and Biostatistics, Istituto Superiore di Sanità,
Rome, Italy

Seidell, Jacob C.
National Institute of Public Health and Environmental Protection, Antonie van
Leeuwenhoeklaan 9, 3720 BA, Bilthoven, The Netherlands

Smit, Henriette A.
National Institute of Public Health and Environmental Protection, Antonie van
Leeuwenhoeklaan 9, 3720 BA, Bilthoven, The Netherlands

Sprafka, J. Michael
Division of Epidemiology, School of Public Health, University of Minnesota, 1300 S. 2nd St., Suite 300, Minneapolis, MN 55454, USA

Stamler, Jeremiah
Department of Preventive Medicine, Northwestern University Medical School, 680 North Lake Shore Drive, Suite 1102, Chicago, IL 60611, USA

Tashiro, Hiromi
The Third Department of Medicine, Kurume University School of Medicine, 67 Asahimachi, Kurume, 830 Japan

Toshima, Hironori
The Third Department of Medicine, Kurume University School of Medicine, 67 Asahimachi, Kurume, 830 Japan

Tsuruta, Makoto
The Third Department of Medicine, Kurume University School of Medicine, 67 Asahimachi, Kurume, 830 Japan

Tuomilehto, Jaakko
Department of Epidemiology and Health Promotion, National Public Health Institute, SF-00510 Helsinki, Finland

Uutela, Antti
Department of Social Psychology, University of Helsinki, SF-00510 Helsinki, Finland

Valkonen, Tapani
Department of Sociology, University of Helsinki, SF-00510 Helsinki, Finland

van Leer, Edith M.
National Institute of Public Health and Environmental Protection, Antonie van Leeuwenhoeklaan 9, 3720 BA, Bilthoven, The Netherlands

Vartiainen, Erkki
Department of Epidemiology and Health Promotion, National Public Health Institute, SF-00510 Helsinki, Finland

Verschuren, W.M. Monique
National Institute of Public Health and Environmental Protection, Antonie van Leeuwenhoeklaan 9, 3720 BA, Bilthoven, The Netherlands

Vukotić, Milija R.
Institute for Cardiovascular Diseases, University Clinical Center, Koste Todorovica 8, 11000 Belgrade, Yugoslavia

Part 1
Overview of the Seven Countries Study

A Brief Personal History of the Seven Countries Study

ANCEL KEYS

Our adventures together began when we wanted to see if an international team could make prospective studies on samples of men in different countries. We made trials in southern Italy and on the island of Crete and discovered mistakes we needed to avoid.

The Seven Countries Study began in 1958 with entry examinations of samples of men in the United States, in Yugoslavia, and here in Japan. That was 35 years ago. Some of you here shared in those adventures. Alas, some of our companions are gone; "they went away," as they say in Italy. But we do not forget Henry Taylor, Paul White, Bozidar Djordjevic, F.S.P. van Buchem, Vittorio Puddu, or Noboru Kimura. We are here in Japan because Noboru Kimura started the work in Japan and continued to direct the prospective studies in Tanushimaru and Ushibuka until an unkind fate took him away.

For me, and I think for most of you, the greatest adventure was living and working with colleagues from other countries and with different backgrounds. Those were rich experiences. Sometimes we had arguments, but never quarrels; we were, and still are, good friends, united in the search for facts to enlighten medical science.

Some of us will recall the adventure of driving on narrow, rocky roads to the villages in Crete. We recall the adventure of working peacefully in Yugoslavia with no signs of animosity among Moslems, Christians, and Communist non-believers; the evil of "ethnic cleansing" is a new horror. It was an adventure to sample the cuisines of the different countries where we worked. For many of us it was an adventure to meet at Anacapri in 1981 and travel by hydrofoil to our region of the Cilento. I hope all of you will tell us about your personal adventures in the Seven Countries work.

Japan, Noboru Kimura, Tanushimaru, and Ushibuka

A week before the 1954 World Congress of Cardiology in Washington, D.C., a Japanese gentleman arrived at Stadium Gate 27 of the University of Minnesota carrying a large brown suitcase. I did not know him but he introduced himself

3

as Dr. Noboru Kimura, Professor of Medicine at the Kurume University Medical School, Japan. He said he had come to get help with classifying electrocardiograms—and opened the suitcase! It was full of electrocardiograms, a thousand he said, and he wanted to report on them at the forthcoming congress. I promptly disclaimed any suggestion that I was expert in regard to ECGs and called in our expert, Dr. Ernst Simonson, who helped classify the material.

Noboru Kimura asked at length what work I was doing, why, and how. He knew I was concerned about the incidence of coronary heart disease, and said it was very rare in his experience. We agreed it would be good to examine the situation in Japan. In 1955 I wrote to Kimura that I would plan to look with him into coronary heart disease and risk factors among Japanese men. He was enthusiastic about my proposal of visiting Japan, and then Dr. Paul White said he would also like to take part in the work. I was also interested in Japanese living outside Japan, so I wrote to Dr. Nils Larsen about examining Japanese in Honolulu. He said he would be glad to arrange for us to work in the Japanese Kuakini Hospital and would bring healthy Japanese men for us to examine. Everyone agreed on the timetable for 1956, Margaret put in order the equipment for measuring serum cholesterol and we, together with Brian Bronte-Stewart, took off for Hawaii. Nils Larsen met us at the airport in Honolulu. There were flowers everywhere and all of us, especially Margaret, were draped with leis; Margaret's lei was full of orchids. Nils Larsen had made all arrangements for us to work at the Kuakini Hospital, laboratory space for Margaret to measure serum cholesterol, a room for examining healthy Japanese men living in Honolulu and those working in two sugar plantations. Three days of rest, entertainment, and sightseeing and we were ready for work The hospital was "first class," and doctors and staff did everything to help our survey.

When Dr. Paul White arrived, he checked patients, examined hospital records, and talked with the local doctors. Coronary patients were uncommon but occasionally were admitted to the hospital. Margaret found that serum cholesterol levels were low. We worked until the last moment before taking off for Japan. As our plane departed, we saw the famous beaches in the sunshine below and regretted we had not had more time to enjoy them.

In 1956, airplanes were slow and limited in fuel capacity, so from Honolulu en route to Japan we stopped overnight at Wake Island. At Tokyo we were met by a man holding up a sign: "WELCOME DR. KEYS." He introduced himself as Dr. Sasamoto, a colleague of Noboru Kimura, and took us to a hotel, saying he would see us the next morning. Our hotel bedroom was spacious and clean, but entirely without beds. In strictly Japanese hotels, a mat (*futon*) is brought in to sleep on the matted padded floor (*tatami*). Dinner was in the hotel restaurant where no one had a word of English. We knew the word *sukiyaki*, said "sukiyaki" to the waiter, and he nodded his head. It was very good.

We were impressed that a Japanese dinner is completely different from Chinese. Even the rice is different, sticky in Japanese but not in Chinese meals. We wondered if they ate sticky rice in Japan because it is easier to eat with chopsticks; you can easily pick up a ball of sticky rice with chopsticks. Eating Chinese rice, the bowl is brought up to the mouth and the rice shoved in with chopsticks.

The next day, Dr. Sasamoto took us sightseeing to several museums and then to visit the hospital at Keio University. We were astonished at the untidiness everywhere in the hospital at that time. An excellent Chinese dinner that evening was the first indication that Japanese and their guests might be treated to Chinese rather than Japanese food. We suspect that Japanese people really like Chinese food but cling to their own cuisine to distinguish themselves.

In the morning, a pleasant surprise was strawberries for breakfast, and on the way to the airport to fly to Osaka we saw wild strawberries growing out of a rock wall. In Tokyo pouring rain alternated with light rain; we were told that is the pattern for March in that part of Japan. In Osaka we were pushed, literally, onto the train to Kyoto for sightseeing. We were told that "pushers" were employed to expedite loading commuting trains.

At the Fukuoka airport, we were met by the Kimuras and by reporters, translators, photographers, and Mr. and Mrs. Midthun, who were attached to the U.S. Information Service. Paul and Ina White arrived a few minutes after we did and we all went to the Kimura home in Kurume for cocktails. Standing there, chatting with glasses in hand, the room suddenly swayed markedly. Margaret said the floor was rising and falling. No, we were not drunk; it was an earthquake, and nobody paid any attention. Such earthquakes are so common there that they hardly cause comment.

After a "business" meeting, we were taken to a Japanese restaurant to eat in proper style—shoes off, sitting on the floor, drinking warm sake out of tiny glasses, eating raw fish and lobster. After a bit we were entertained by geishas in their flowered kimonos, who poured sake, danced, and had us all playing what they call the "baseball game," one at a time on stage. The next day was Easter Sunday, rainy, and we went to a Christian church. The sermon was all in Japanese but they sang "Christ the Lord Is Risen Today." Later in the day we set up the laboratory equipment and the electrocardiograph machine and again were appalled at the disorder. Margaret climbed up on the benches to wash the windows.

While I was working with the medical team examining some local workers at Noboru's Department of Medicine at the Medical School, Margaret was taken to see a class in flower arranging. One formality was stressed: never arrange with four flowers. The Japanese tend to be more sensitive to beauty in color and graceful form than most Westerners. Visiting Japanese homes and purely Japanese hotels a sense of beauty was shown in spacious bedrooms, the only furniture in sight being a low table of fine wood; mats are brought in for sleeping. The quiet elegance of such bedrooms did not prepare one for a breakfast of dried seaweed, pickles, fish custard, cold rice, and tea!

It was springtime, and going to a park we found an immense crowd admiring the cherry blossoms, with music in the background and dancing girls performing. A land of contrasts. Visiting a mining town, it was surprising to see that all the miners coming from work were very clean. We were taken to a concert by the Vienna Philharmonic Orchestra. The hall with 1000 seats was full, with many standing to listen to renditions of Schubert and Mendelssohn. The audience was very responsive.

Our 1956 visit to Japan involved surveys of diet, blood cholesterol, electrocardiograms, anthropometric measurements, and demonstrations of methods used. All this was only an exploration. The men we examined were not a particular sample of any kind of men, but we only wanted to get a general idea of how to work in a study in Japan.

In 1958, Noboru Kimura and his staff started a prospective study on men aged 40 to 59 at the farming village of Tanushimaru, conveniently close to the Kurume Medical School and Kimura's Department of Medicine. None of us at the University of Minnesota took part in the examinations or measurements, and there were some discrepancies in the procedure and methods. Later reexaminations of the men of Tanushimaru conformed strictly to the procedures and methods of the other cohorts of the Seven Countries Study, but some data from the 1958 examinations are not comparable to the data in the other cohorts.

In 1960, Noboru Kimura started a prospective study on the men of Ushibuka, a fishermen's village at the southern tip of the island of Kyushu. The 502 men of Ushibuka make a contrast with the 508 men of Tanushimaru: fishermen versus farmers. The fishing ships from Ushibuka go clear across the Pacific Ocean to fish off the shores of Chile and Peru. The round trip takes 3 weeks or more, the fishermen subsisting on a diet of raw fish, rice, and tea. In the long-time follow-up, the men of Ushibuka have differed little in mortality from the men of Tanushimaru; the men of both areas rarely developed coronary heart disease.

Both in Tanushimaru and Ushibuka the men tended to be heavy smokers. The average percentage of smokers in the two cohorts and the average number of cigarettes smoked daily were higher than in any of the other cohorts in the Seven Countries Study. It was surprising, then, to find that the habit of smoking was not found to be a major risk factor for premature death in the 25-year follow-up. One possible reason for the lack of a relation between smoking and mortality may be in the kind of cigarettes smoked. The tobacco used was grown in the southernmost island of Japan, the variety of tobacco being the same as in the United States. However, additives in the manufacture of the cigarettes were not used as in the United States; nothing is added to the tobacco to keep it burning when the smoke is not being inhaled from the lighted cigarette. The cure of the tobacco and the paper in the Japanese cigarettes may also differ from that in the United States. Recently, the cigarettes smoked in Japan tend to be more like American cigarettes but, as yet, there are no good data on a changed relation of mortality to smoking in Japan.

The second place for our prospective study in Japan is Ushibuka, a fishing village at the tip of a long peninsula of Kyushu. It was not easy to get there. The easiest route in the period of the initial examinations and early follow-up was to go by train from Fukuoka to Minamata and then by ferry across the strait to Ushibuka. (No doubt it is easier now, flying to Minamata for the first part of the travel.) When Margaret and I visited Ushibuka, the crossing from Minamata was in a tiny ferry boat, sitting on deck and hanging on. The alternative was a microscopic, airless cabin with no window. Our arrival at Ushibuka was greeted effusively, and an elaborate luncheon was provided at table with about 20 doctors and officials. But first we must have the honorable hot bath. We were escorted to a room with a steaming tub of water, more like a small shallow swimming pool, with ample room for two persons, and were provided with very small towels to use after being properly soaked in the hot water. We had to go through with it. Margaret was upset because the steam made a mess of her hair. We could not get really dry with the tiny towels. When we got out, dressed, and went into the room to have lunch, there were the Japanese, sitting at the table, waiting for us all the time.

Our experience with Japanese and their customs is dated from the mid-1950s to the end of the 1960s. The Japanese and their customs in the 1990s are different, reflecting a changed economy and the effects of emerging from relative isolation to a new place in the world, exposed to the impact of seeing, hearing, and reading about other populations, other cultures. This is a time of change in all peoples; the Japanese are perhaps changing more than people in the other areas in the Seven Countries Study. The distribution of deaths by cause as indicated in the vital statistics is changing, with far fewer deaths from infectious disease. But today I remember Japan and the Japanese as they were. Noboru Kimura is gone, but he and the Japan we experienced are still vividly in mind.

Acknowledgments. I want particularly to acknowledge the long and faithful service to this study of Mrs. Rose Hilk in data entry, programming, and analysis, and of John Vilandre in computational support, both at the University of Minnesota Coordinating Center.

The Seven Countries Study:
A Historic Adventure in Science

HENRY BLACKBURN

Key words. Cardiovascular disease epidemiology—Seven Countries Study

Introduction

The Seven Countries Study (SCS) has become a classic in science for its pioneering effort in cardiovascular disease (CVD) epidemiology and for its powerful lesson to science: that mass phenomena determine the population rates and the preventive strategies of CVD. The idea of the SCS arose in various forms in the minds of imaginative individuals capable of integrating laboratory, clinical, and population evidence. The study was given substance and direction by its leader, our colleague Ancel Keys.

The SCS was first to make systematic comparisons of CVD rates and characteristics of risk in contrasting cultures. It was first to combine cross-sectional surveys with long-term follow-up among cohorts. It was first to compute population (ecologic) correlations between lifestyle and risk factors and between risk factors and disease, and their *changes* over time. It was first to apply multivariate regression coefficients derived in one population to findings in men of the same age in another. Thereby it demonstrated both that the major CVD risk factors are universal and that the *force* of a risk factor differs among contrasting populations, and among populations compared to individuals. The SCS has had a major influence on the thinking, methods and research into the causes and prevention of CVD, and on the public health.

Keys and collaborators hypothesized that differences in population rates of CVD, and individual risk within populations, were related to mode of life and risk factors, including composition of the diet. To examine this hypothesis, following pilot studies in Finland, Italy, and Crete in 1957, formal cross-sectional surveys were conducted, starting in 1958, among samples of men aged 40–59, in seven countries contrasting in composition of the diet and in purported heart disease rates: Yugoslavia, Italy, Greece, the Netherlands, Finland, Japan, and the United States. Baseline survey participants were entered into cohorts and both the diseased and disease-free were followed for 30 years in most areas. The study was unique for its time, with "adequately-sized" "chunk" samples in 18 areas as the cohorts, with standardized risk factor and disease measurements, training of teams, and central coding and analysis of data. The SCS became the prototypical population comparison study, made across a wide range of diet and disease experience.

In this anniversary symposium, we review the grand story of the SCS [3]. We summarize the early and ongoing contributions of its leaders and participants during 35 years of a unique scientific collaboration and shared personal adventure.

A Brief Background and History

The Seven Countries Study developed out of a rich set of observations made by a number of clinicians and investigators. It emerged in embryonic form in each of the seven countries. There was, in the late 1950s, a readiness for the ideas, along with preparedness for effective research among disciplines and across cultures. Ancel Keys and the Minnesota group had participated in physiological studies during and after World War II, had found the importance of nutrition and lifestyle in human biology (which they called physiological hygiene), and had recognized early that cardiovascular diseases were a major new public health concern. Keys and colleagues were also prepared with quantitative thinking and computational skills, able to link ideas, bridge disciplines, and apply methods appropriate to the scientific question. Taylor and colleagues at Minnesota in 1957 initiated U.S. efforts of the SCS in a study of CVD rates in railway occupations that required different levels of physical activity. At the same time, researchers in several parts of the world were examining similar issues: Karvonen and the Finnish group, Fidanza and Puddu of the Italian group, Buzina and Djordjevic and the two Yugoslavian groups, Aravanis and Dontas and the Greek group, Kimura and Toshima and the Japanese group, and Dalderup and colleagues of the Dutch group. Each had already begun explorations of population phenomena in CVD, testing hypotheses about the causal role of diet, physical activity, and lifestyle. Back in Minnesota, Keys, Grande, and Anderson also made crucial systematic metabolic experiments on the precise serum cholesterol effects of diet changes. Essential to the whole were the observations of Paul Dudley White and Noboru Kimura, who put into bold and simple terms the differences in CVD frequency and arterial pathology seen around the world. Meetings between all of these remarkable people were stimulated by Ancel Keys; the ideas for collaborative research rapidly took hold, and active work began. Pilot studies with the Finns in 1956 and the Italians and Greeks in 1957 demonstrated feasibility of the SCS in the field. The central coordinating grant to Professor Keys from the U.S. National Institutes of Health (NIH) allowed the definitive cohort surveys to begin in Yugoslavia in 1958, while the U.S. Railroad Study had proceeded in 1957 under a separate grant to Henry Taylor.

Fortunately for the SCS, national Heart Foundations and other groups were ready to support the early phases of these activities. The U.S. Railroad Study profited from the support of the new National Heart Institute (NHI). Ancel Keys, of course, played the central role of putting all the ideas together in a clear proposal to the NHI for collaborative research among the seven countries. He had the international contacts, the vision, and the experience to move this major project forward.

Finally, the special experience and knowledge of each of the SCS principal investigators about their professional fields, and about the geography and culture of their lands, along with their clinical contacts and political clout, enabled the whole SCS operation to be put in motion. The central NIH budget at the time was only about U.S. $25 000 per year per center, so the fund-raising talents of all the princepal investigators were quickly developed!

As remarkable as these beginnings was the later emergence of leadership in the SCS, from various places, where and when it was needed. Ancel Keys' leadership was essential to organize the study, prepare the initial collaborative proposal, and, over the years, bring out the three major monographs: the 1967 *Acta Medica Scandinavia* supplement, the 1970 *Circulation* supplement, and the 1980 Oxford Press monograph. Each of these efforts was a tour de force that brought the diverse findings together in a way that no other investigator or editorial board could have done as cogently and effectively. But other leadership appeared when the SCS came under its greatest threat—the central grant expired in the late 1960s, and soon after Dr. Keys retired and his base of operations was constrained. This was paralleled by the necessarily intense preoccupation in Minnesota with new activities to assure the survival and growth of the Laboratory of Physiological Hygiene, then and still a largely self-supporting academic institution. Thus, in the late 1960s much of the SCS energy, data collection, and coordinating responsibility was shifted to the capable hands of Alessandro Menotti and the Rome center.

Since then an important new axis of leadership has developed between the Netherlands, Rome, and Finland, with a rich collegial sharing of ideas, initiatives, and new data collection for new researches. The SCS owes much to the enterprise of Kromhout, Menotti, and Nissinen in this development. Daan Kromhout has taken the initiative in extending the dietary analyses and in sponsoring a major historical monograph on the SCS to be unveiled at this conference. Hironori Toshima has organized and funded this remarkable anniversary meeting, an intellectually stimulating and charming social occasion, along with publication of the scientific proceedings.

In addition to the long list of SCS "firsts" as detailed in these presentations and publications, the study continues to redefine its mission and hypotheses. For example, there is every evidence of continued success in the long-term follow-up of survival in the cohorts. Dr. Keys continues to study longevity related to characteristics at entry. And researches by the several investigators move to explain further the large differences in population CVD rates, and the individual differences in risk with respect to differences, *and to changes over time*, in diet and other risk factors.

Of course, there are problems. The Seven Countries Study has a relatively small number of units to compare, with few degrees of freedom for the ecological correlations, and making these correlations at all was early criticized. Some have also criticized the selection of the different geographic areas, the varied occupational composition of the populations compared, and the obvious technical limitations of measurement and classification across areas by national teams, often under difficult field survey conditions. It is true that improvements have been made in the configuration of populations for such internal and international comparisons, by random selection of greater numbers of units, and other means. But the SCS was not only "state of the art" for its time; it was bold and foresighted in its concepts and thrust. And, as we increasingly realize today, the ecological associations of habitual diet, other risk factors, and population rates of disease, in themselves weak sources of causal inference, are nevertheless, with strong congruent evidence from the laboratory and clinic, valuable indicators of the forces underlying mass diseases. When the evidence is consistent, the population correlations may indicate the major determinants of different population rates of disease.

Results and Conclusions

The SCS, perhaps more than any other scientific study in history, has directed attention to the causes of *population* rates of disease, in contrast to the causes of individual risk. It has documented large population differences in disease rates and in the average risk factor levels related to the different rates. It has demonstrated the degree to which composition of the diet, particularly in saturated fatty acids, and mean population serum cholesterol levels predict present and future population rates of coronary heart disease.

The regressions derived from the ecological correlations of risk and CVD in the SCS as a whole have provided the "rule," while departure from this prediction line has disclosed important "exceptions," such as the excess of CVD in East Finland and the paradox of Crete, with high-fat diet, mid-range serum cholesterol levels, and low CHD rates. These findings, in turn, have provided impetus to researches on mass CVD determinants other than saturated fatty acids, including omega-3 and monounsaturated fatty acids, fibers, and recently, antioxidants. Finally, the SCS has laid a major foundation stone on which has been built new preventive researches and programs, extending from the laboratory to the clinic and back to entire populations.

We celebrate here a great scientific adventure, an adventure in new ideas and methods, an adventure in collegiality and in organization for effective collaboration, and an adventure which has had the greatest influence on thinking, on practice, and on policy in cardiovascular disease medicine and on the public health. Let the celebration continue!

Discussion

M. Karvonen: Thank you very much, Henry. You explained everything! If any of you still have questions, just ask Henry after this meeting. Never has such a global undertaking been condensed so perfectly.

Part 2
Update on the Seven Countries Study

Risk Factors and Mortality Patterns in the Seven Countries Study

ALESSANDRO MENOTTI and FULVIA SECCARECCIA

Summary. The 16 cohorts of the Seven Countries Study were enrolled in the United States (1); in Finland (2); in the Netherlands (1); in Italy (3), in Croatia, former Yugoslavia (2); in Serbia, former Yugoslavia (3); in Greece (2); and in Japan (2), for a total of more than 12000 men aged 40 to 59 years at entry. The pattern of the mean levels of four cardiovascular risk factors in each cohort (systolic blood pressure, serum cholesterol, body mass index, and smoking habits) was related to the pattern of mortality in 10 and 25 years, taking into account five causes of death (coronary heart disease, CHD; strokes, STR; lung cancer, LUCA; other cancers, OCA; all other causes of death, OTH). Simple linear correlation, multiple linear regression, and canonical correlation showed that the overall dominant cause of death was CHD, which also showed the largest variability among cohorts. Out of the four risk factors, serum cholesterol showed the largest variability at baseline and the largest change during the first 10 years of follow-up. In all types of analysis, the main population (ecologic) correlations found were of mean serum cholesterol to rates of CHD, of cigarette smoking to LUCA, and of cholesterol and blood pressure (negative) to STR rates.

Key words. Seven Countries—Risk factors—Mortality—Coronary heart disease

Introduction

The Seven Countries Study is an epidemiological enterprise starting in the late 1950s, which tried to answer basic questions on the etiology of cardiovascular and coronary heart disease rates in populations [1]. They were: (1) whether real differences existed in incidence and mortality from cardiovascular, and mainly coronary, heart disease among contrasting populations; (2) whether differences, if any, could be explained by general characteristics or lifestyles of the populations; and (3) whether individual characteristics within different populations predict the individual risk of future morbid or fatal events.

These basic questions were substantially answered after 10 years of follow-up and were reported in major monographs and other publications [1–6]. Other questions were suggested by the available data accumulated in the 25-year follow-up. A compelling new question was whether the overall pattern of risk factors and their change could be related, in cohort comparisons, to the pattern of mortality from the several main causes of death.

This analysis attempts to relate the risk factor pattern with the mortality pattern, exploiting the three survey examinations conducted in the field for measurement of risk factors (at 0, 5, and 10 years) and the 25-year mortality experience.

Materials and Methods

The Seven Countries Study was conducted in 16 cohorts of men aged 40 to 59 years, in seven different countries. Details on enrollment were given elsewhere [1,2,4]. Altogether there were 11 "chunk" samples of men residing in defined rural areas in Finland (East and West Finland), in Italy (Crevalcore and Montegiorgio), in former Yugoslavia (Dalmatia and Slavonia in Croatia, Velika Krsna in Serbia), in Greece (the islands of Crete and Corfu), and in Japan (Tanushimaru and Ushibuka); samples of railroad employees in defined occupational jobs and defined areas (one in the United States and one in Italy); a statistical sample of men in Zutphen, a small commercial town in the Netherlands; an occupational group of men in an agroindustrial cooperative in Zrenjanin, Serbia, former Yugoslavia; and a sample of university professors in Belgrade, former Yugoslavia. The size of the samples ranged from about 500 to 2500 subjects, for a total of 12761 men examined at entry, with an overall average participation rate of about 90%. The field surveys at years 0, 5, and 10 were centrally coordinated and performed by international teams of physicians, nurses, technicians, and dietitians who collected data in a uniform and standardized way following a common protocol [1,2,4]. Measurements included anthropometric, biochemical, biophysical, social, behavioral, nutritional, and clinical characteristics. Other examinations at longer follow-up intervals were organized in a scattered and not always coordinated way and will not be taken into account in this report.

For the purpose of this analysis, only a few measurements are considered, corresponding to classical risk factors for cardiovascular diseases. Age, in years, was rounded off at the nearest birthday; height, in centimeters, and weight, in kilograms, were taken in light underwear and without shoes, following the technique later described by the World Health Organization Manual on Cardiovascular Survey Methods [7] (from now on called the WHO Manual). Height and weight were used to compute body mass index (kg/m^2). Blood pressure (mmHg) was measured in the right arm, in the supine position, at the end of the clinical examination by trained and tested physicians using a standard mercury sphygmomanometer and following the procedure described in the WHO Manual [7]. Readings were made to the nearest 2 mmHg. Diastolic blood pressure was recorded both as fourth and fifth phase of the Korotkoff sounds. Two consecutive measurements were taken 2 min apart. For the purpose of this analysis, diastolic blood pressure was ignored and systolic blood pressure was defined as the average of two consecutive measurements. Serum cholesterol was measured on casual blood samples following the Abell–Kendall technique as modified by Anderson and Keys [8]. Smoking habits were determined from a questionnaire, and the indicator employed for this analysis was the prevalence of smokers in the several population samples.

The repeated field examinations allowed the measurement of incidence of major cardiovascular diseases, but this analysis is confined to deaths during 25 years follow-up.

The mortality data were collected systematically from periodic visits on the spot. The final diagnostic cause of death was adjudicated by a single reviewer to whom information was made available on the official death certification (seldom used alone); on medical history collected from interviewing doctors, from relatives of the dead persons, and other witnesses; and by abstracting clinical records. The basic coding used the eighth revision of the WHO International Classification of Diseases (WHO-ICD) [9]; internal codes were employed for a more compact classification [2]. Age standardization of death rates was made taking as a reference population the quinquennial age distribution of the whole Seven Countries Study population at entry.

The analysis reported here was based on comparisons between cohorts, ignoring single individuals. Each one of the 16 cohorts represented one statistical unit and each was therefore characterized by mean levels of the chosen risk factors and by age-standardized death rates. The latter were limited to a small number of diagnostic subgroups—coronary heart disease (CHD), strokes (STR), lung cancer (LUCA), other cancers (OCA), and all other causes of death (OTH). The analysis was run along three different lines: (1) computation of simple linear correlation of rates for each cause of death on mean population values for each risk factor (measured at baseline) as related to 10 and 25 years of follow-up; (2) computation of the multiple linear regression and ecologic correlation of each cause of death on all the chosen risk factors (measured at baseline) as related to 10 and 25 years of follow-up; and (3) computation of the canonical correlation that related the whole set of risk factors to the whole set of death rates. This analysis was broken down into two parts: (1) computation of the canonical correlation relating the baseline risk factor levels to the death rate groupings, and separately for cumulative mortality data of 5, 10, 15, 20, and 25 years follow-up (descriptive and tabulated details are limited, however, to data corresponding to follow-ups of 10 and 25 years only), and (2) computation of the canonical correlation for the 15 years following the first 10 (death rates from year 10 to year 25 of follow-up). In this case two analyses were made, one taking into account the relationship of baseline risk factor levels to the delayed 10- to 25-year mortality, and the other by adding, as covariates, the population risk factor changes that occurred in 10 years (levels of year 10 minus levels of year 0, called Deltas), in order to investigate the role of population changes in delayed mortality experience. The Deltas for the U.S. cohort used the 5-year risk factor measurements, since the 10-year reexamination was not performed.

Because the canonical correlation analysis method is not well known [10], a few notes on its meaning are given here. It is an extension of multiple linear correlation and regression, where, on the y axis (dependent variable), more than one variable is included. Similar to the traditional multiple linear regression, many xs are present (independent variables). Usually the xs represent the hypothesized causes, whereas ys represent the supposed effects. The technique finds several linear combinations of the xs and the same number of linear combinations of the ys in such a way that these linear combinations best express the correlation between the two sets. Those linear combinations are called the canonical variables (V_i for the linear combination of the xs and U_i for the linear combination of the ys). The correlation between the corresponding pairs of canonical variables is called the canonical correlation. In the analysis, the mean of each variable is subtracted from the original data so that the sample means of the x and y variables are zero. For each variable in the two sets (the xs and the ys), a coefficient is estimated and, to compare them with each other, their standardized values are adopted (the coefficient divided by the standard deviation of the original variable). The canonical correlation is expressed as a simple linear correlation coefficient and its square is called the eigenvalue. It should be recalled that the canonical correlation coefficient is larger than any simple correlation coefficient between any x and any y variables. A number of derived measurements and tests are also produced, but they will be introduced and defined when used in the text. A small number of canonical correlations can be computed after the first, but this analysis will be confined to the first canonical correlation only.

Results

Risk Factors and Death Rates

Table 1 shows the means of the cohorts for the four major risk factors in the 16 cohorts as measured at entry, with their variability. The coefficients of variation indicate that a relatively large variability exists for serum cholesterol and for prevalence of smokers, whereas little variation was shown for systolic blood pressure and body mass index. The highest levels in blood cholesterol were found in the Finnish cohorts, the lowest in two of the Serbian cohorts and in Japan. The highest levels of blood pressure were in East Finland and Crevalcore, Italy, the lowest in Velika Krsna, Serbia. Smoking habit was highly prevalent among the Japanese and Dutch men and much less in Belgrade and Velika Krsna, Serbia. Body mass index was rather high in the Rome railroad men and in the Belgrade professors, and rather low among men in Japan and in Crete and Dalmatia.

Table 1. Seven Countries Study: Entry mean levels of four risk factors in 16 cohorts, and their variability among cohorts.

	Mean	S.D.	Minimum	Maximum	Coefficient of variation
Systolic blood pressure (mmHg)	138.4	5.0	131.4	148.4	0.03
Cholesterol level (mg/dl)	204.8	32.1	160.1	266.2	0.16
Body mass index (kg/m^2)	24.0	1.51	21.8	26.6	0.06
Smokers (%)	61	9	44	78	14

S.D., standard deviation.

Table 2. Seven Countries Study: Correlation matrix of entry mean levels of four major risk factors among 16 cohorts.

	SBP	CHOL	BMI	SMOKE
SBP	1.00			
CHOL	0.67*	1.00		
BMI	0.30	0.35	1.00	
SMOKE	0.38	−0.01	−0.28	1.00

*$P < 0.01$.
SBP, systolic blood pressure; CHOL, serum cholesterol level; BMI, body mass index; SMOKE, smoking habits.

The correlation matrix among all possible pairs of risk factors (Table 2) shows a relatively high relationship among all the possible pairs except between cholesterol and smokers' prevalence. However, only the correlation between systolic blood pressure and cholesterol ($r = 0.67$) is statistically significant.

Table 3 gives an overall picture of death rates (means among the 16 cohorts) with their variability. All of the five diagnostic groupings exhibit relatively large variation coefficients, but those of CHD and LUCA largely exceed all the others. The highest rates of CHD were found in Finland, in the U.S. railroad sample, and in Zutphen, the Netherlands; the lowest were observed in Japan and Crete. On the other hand, the cohorts with the greatest burden of strokes were Zrenjanin in Serbia, Slavonia in Croatia, and Ushibuka in Japan, whereas this condition was relatively rare in Belgrade and in the Finnish cohorts. Lung cancer was rather common in men in East Finland and in Zutphen, the Netherlands, and much less in Japan and in the three Serbian cohorts. Other cancers showed peaks in Ushibuka, Japan, Crevalcore, Italy and Zrenjanin, Serbia and very low levels in Belgrade and Crete. All "other" causes of death were exceedingly frequent in Slavonia (mainly due to tuberculosis) and definitely rare in Belgrade.

The correlation matrix computed for the five major mortality groupings shows a highly positive relationship between CHD and LUCA on one side and

Table 3. Seven Countries Study: Death rates from five major causes, per 1000 in 16 cohorts in 25 years, and their variability among cohorts.

	Mean	S.D.	Minimum	Maximum	Coefficient of variation
Coronary heart disease	134	65	46	288	0.48
Stroke	70	27	36	120	0.39
Lung cancer	31	18	9	73	0.59
Other cancers	93	28	54	156	0.30
Other causes	136	47	49	251	0.35

S.D., standard deviation.

Table 4. Seven Countries Study: Correlation matrix of death rates from five major causes in 25 years among the 16 cohorts.

	CHD	STR	LUCA	OCA	OTH
CHD	1.00				
STR	−0.42	1.00			
LUCA	0.74**	−0.56	1.00		
OCA	−0.32	0.36	−0.28	1.00	
OTH	−0.12	0.73**	−0.31	0.18	1.00

** $P < 0.01$.
CHD, coronary heart disease; STR, strokes; LUCA, lung cancer; OCA, other cancers; OTH, all other causes.

between STR and OTH on the other, whereas a negative significant correlation was found between STR and LUCA (Table 4).

Simple Linear Correlations

The (ecologic) correlation matrix between entry levels of risk factors and the major diagnostic groupings shows similar findings for the 10-year and 25-year mortality data (Tables 5 and 6). In particular, CHD rates in the population are highly correlated with mean blood pressure and cholesterol levels; STR is negatively correlated with systolic blood pressure, cholesterol, and body mass index; LUCA is directly correlated with blood pressure and cholesterol; OCA is inversely correlated with cholesterol and directly with smoker prevalence; OTH is negatively correlated with body mass index. In most cases, except for CHD, the correlations are stronger in the 25-year matrix than in the 10-year one.

Some of these ecologic correlations are biologically plausible (e.g., population cholesterol levels *vs* CHD rates), some are of dubious causal interpretation (cholesterol and blood pressure *vs* LUCA), and some are even paradoxical, such as the inverse relationship of mean blood pressure to STR rates. The

Table 5. Seven Countries Study: Linear correlation coefficients of five major causes of death in 10 years on entry mean levels of four risk factors.

	CHD	STR	LUCA	OCA	OTH
Systolic blood pressure	0.71**	−0.31	0.79***	0.10	−0.04
Cholesterol	0.82***	−0.54*	0.71**	−0.30	−0.33
Body mass index	0.33	−0.10	0.23	−0.18	−0.46
Smokers (%)	0.17	0.23	0.39	0.62**	0.13

* $P < 0.05$; ** $P < 0.01$; *** $P < 0.001$.

CHD, coronary heart disease; STR, strokes; LUCA, lung cancer; OCA, other cancers; OTH, all other causes.

Table 6. Seven Countries Study: Linear correlation coefficients of five major causes of death in 25 years on entry mean levels of four risk factors.

	CHD	STR	LUCA	OCA	OTH
Systolic blood pressure	0.59*	−0.55*	0.75***	0.02	−0.14
Cholesterol	0.73**	−0.78***	0.75***	−0.52*	−0.38
Body mass index	0.36	−0.51*	0.11	−0.09	−0.50*
Smokers (%)	0.06	0.12	0.37	0.57*	0.05

* $P < 0.05$; ** $P < 0.01$; *** $P < 0.001$.

CHD, coronary heart disease; STR, strokes; LUCA, lung cancer; OCA, other cancers; OTH, all other causes.

latest result found (−0.55 in the 25-year follow-up) was reconsidered by computing the partial correlation coefficient of blood pressure *vs* STR, holding cholesterol constant, and was close to zero (−0.06). On the other hand, the partial correlation coefficient of cholesterol *vs* STR (with blood pressure kept constant) remained high and significant (−0.66).

Multiple Linear Correlation

A second step in the analysis concerned the computation of multiple linear regression equations and correlations between each of the mortality endpoints in 10 and 25 years and the four risk factors. A summary is given in Table 7, where only the squared multiple correlation coefficients are shown. The highest *r* square values in the 10-year follow-up were those for CHD and LUCA (both statistically significant), whereas in the 25-year experience, all the *P* values were significant except that for OTH. This means that single diagnostic groups are predicted by the small set of risk factors (mainly at the 25-year follow-up), although only a few regression coefficients are statistically significant. In the 10-year follow-up equations, cholesterol was significantly related to CHD and smokers' prevalence to OCA; in the 25-year follow-up equations, cholesterol was significantly and negatively correlated with STR and OCA and positively correlated with LUCA.

Table 7. Seven Countries Study: Squared multiple correlation of each major cause of death in 10 and 25 years is on four major risk factors, as derived by a series of multiple linear regression equations.

	10 Years		25 Years	
	r squared	P	r squared	P
CHD	0.728	0.004	0.560	0.044
STR	0.385	0.214	0.681	0.008
LUCA	0.728	0.004	0.722	0.002
OCA	0.482	0.097	0.687	0.007
OTH	0.351	0.270	0.387	0.210

CHD, coronary heart disease; STR, strokes; LUCA, lung cancer; OCA, other cancers; OTH, all other causes.

Canonical Analysis

The first part of the analysis, the canonical correlation, relates the entry mean levels of the four risk factors with the overall 10-year mortality experience. The analysis is summarized in a composite tabulation (Table 8) reporting the standardized coefficients for the x and y variables (and their canonical loadings), plus the canonical correlation coefficient, the canonical eigenvalue, and probability by the Bartlett's test. The highest standardized coefficients for the "causal" variables are, in rank order, those for cholesterol, blood pressure, and smoking habits, whereas the highest standardized coefficients of the "effect" variables are those of CHD and LUCA, with a low (negative) coefficient for STR. This means that the higher the population values of the first three variables, the higher the death rates from CHD and LUCA and the lower the death rates from STR. This is partly reflected also in the canonical loadings, which represent the linear correlation coefficients between the canonical variables and the original variables in each of the two sets. This represents the contribution of the original x and y variables in the construction of the canonical variables V_i and U_i, respectively. In other words, a population sample with high levels of cholesterol, blood pressure, and smoking habits would score high on canonical variable V (possible causes), and similarly a population with high CHD and LUCA and low STR death rates will score high on canonical variable U (possible effects). As an example, the cohorts scoring highest in both V and U canonical variables were East Finland and Zutphen, whereas those exhibiting the smallest values were the Serbian ones, Dalmatia in Croatia, and Montegiorgio in Italy. All this reflected relatively high levels of cholesterol, blood pressure, and smoking habits in the first two cohorts together with high rates of CHD and LUCA and low rates of STR. The reverse was true for the latter four cohorts, which scored very low in the two canonical variables.

Table 8. Seven Countries Study: Canonical correlation analysis between four risk factors at baseline and five endpoints in 10 years of follow-up.

	Standardized canonical coefficients	Canonical loadings
Variables X		
Systolic blood pressure (mmHg)	0.500	0.924
Cholesterol (mg/dl)	0.523	0.823
Body mass index (kg/m^2)	−0.081	0.180
Smokers (%)	0.261	0.469
Variables Y		
Coronary heart disease	0.529	0.849
Strokes	−0.394	−0.392
Lung cancer	0.429	0.897
Other cancers	0.410	0.076
All other causes	0.147	−0.132
Canonical correlation coefficient	0.946	
Canonical eigenvalue	0.894	
Bartlett's test P	0.017	

Incidentally, cholesterol and the prevalence of smokers on the x side and CHD and LUCA on the y side were the variables with the highest coefficients of variation around the mean levels computed on the 16 population samples (Tables 1 and 3), whereas the negative relationship between blood pressure and STR was already shown as partially confounded by cholesterol levels. The resulting canonical correlation coefficient and the corresponding eigenvalue are very high, on the order of 0.90. The Bartlett's test, with its P value, is computed on the eigenvalue and it is significant. As an example taken from the 10-year analysis, the two cohorts scoring highest in both V_i and U_i canonical variables were East Finland and Zutphen, whereas those exhibiting the smallest levels were the Serbian ones, Dalmatia, and Montegiorgio. All this reflected relatively high levels of cholesterol, blood pressure, and smoking habits in the two Finnish cohorts and in Zutphen, together with high rates from CHD and lung cancer and low levels of STR. The reverse was true for the cohorts scoring very low in the two canonical variables.

In a second step, the canonical correlation was computed between the baseline levels of the four risk factors and the mortality rates from year 0 to year 25 of follow-up (Table 9). The overall picture was not very different from that observed in the first 10 years. Among x variables the dominant standardized coefficient is that of cholesterol, whereas the dominant coefficients among y variables are those of CHD (positive) and of STR (negative). The level of the canonical correlation coefficient reached the value of 0.950 (eigenvalue 0.902).

A final step was made (Table 10) by considering the delayed mortality that occurred between year 10 and 25 of the follow-up. The canonical correlation

Table 9. Seven Countries Study: Canonical correlation analysis between four risk factors at baseline and five endpoints in 25 years of follow-up.

	Standardized canonical coefficients	Canonical loadings
Variables X		
Systolic blood pressure (mmHg)	0.105	0.571
Cholesterol (mg/dl)	0.861	0.953
Body mass index (kg/m^2)	0.049	0.472
Smokers (%)	−0.318	−0.302
Variables Y		
Coronary heart disease	0.400	0.724
Strokes	−0.794	−0.836
Lung cancer	−0.114	0.647
Other cancers	−0.332	−0.668
All other causes	0.247	−0.405
Canonical correlation coefficient	0.950	
Canonical eigenvalue	0.902	
Bartlett's test P	0.0003	

Table 10. Seven Countries Study: Canonical correlation analysis between four risk factors at baseline and five delayed endpoints (death occurred between years 10 and 25).

	Standardized canonical coefficients	Canonical loadings
Variables X		
Systolic blood pressure (mmHg)	−0.083	0.544
Cholesterol (mg/dl)	0.976	0.968
Body mass index (kg/m^2)	0.120	0.476
Smokers (%)	−0.163	−0.261
Variables Y		
Coronary heart disease	0.298	0.663
Strokes	−0.638	−0.820
Lung cancer	0.030	0.657
Other cancers	−0.417	−0.689
All other causes	0.067	−0.421
Canonical correlation coefficient	0.930	
Canonical eigenvalue	0.866	
Bartlett's test P	0.0013	

relating baseline risk factor levels to the 10- to 25-year mortality rates show that the dominant variable x is cholesterol whereas the y variables with the highest coefficients are STR and OCA (negative) and CHD (positive). This means that high baseline levels of cholesterol are associated with delayed high

Table 11. Seven Countries Study: Canonical correlation analysis between four risk factors at baseline and their changes in 10 years (Delta) versus five delayed endpoints (death occurred between years 10 and 25).

	Standardized canonical coefficients	Canonical loadings
Variables X		
Systolic blood pressure (mmHg)	0.441	−0.248
Cholesterol (mg/dl)	−0.517	−0.459
Body mass index (kg/m^2)	−0.106	−0.521
Smokers (%)	−0.543	−0.038
Delta-systolic BP	0.607	0.353
Delta-cholesterol	−0.969	−0.165
Delta-BMI	0.463	0.050
Delta-smokers	0.617	0.647
Variables Y		
Coronary heart disease	−0.761	−0.553
Strokes	−0.460	0.521
Lung cancer	0.093	−0.496
Other cancers	−0.025	0.140
All other causes	1.116	0.778
Canonical correlation coefficient	0.997	
Canonical eigenvalue	0.993	
Bartlett's test P	0.0000	

CHD rates and delayed low STR and OCA rates. The canonical correlation coefficient was high (0.930).

In the next step (Table 11), we used the same endpoints, but adding to the xs also the 10-year changes (Deltas) of the various risk factors (mean population values at year 10 minus mean values at year 0). In this system, a positive Delta means an increase of the mean level whereas a negative Delta means a decrease. In this analysis, which includes the risk factor changes in the first 10 years as part of the x variables, the canonical correlation coefficient became much higher, with a value of 0.997 (eigenvalue − 0.993) which is very close to 1.0, suggesting that the linear combination of the Vs and the Us is almost perfect.

Interpretation of the details suggests that in a population with low levels of cholesterol, low levels of smoking habits, large increases in blood pressure, large decreases in cholesterol and a relatively small decrease of smokers will produce a high-ranking V_i canonical variable (possible causes) and, on the other hand, will correspond to low levels of CHD, in spite of relatively high levels of blood pressure. Relatively high levels of blood pressure and relatively large increases in blood pressure levels correspond to relatively low rates of STR. Low levels of smoking habits, followed by large increases (actually, by limited decreases) are associated with some excess of lung cancer and a large

Table 12. Seven Countries Study: Summary of canonical analysis of four risk factors versus five causes of death in 16 cohorts.

Risk factors year	Death rates years	Canonical correlation	Canonical eigenvalue	Bartlett's test P
0	0–5	0.935	0.874	0.1202
0	0–10	0.946	0.894	0.0168
0	0–15	0.935	0.874	0.0059
0	0–20	0.959	0.920	0.0003
0	0–25	0.950	0.902	0.0003
0	10–25	0.930	0.866	0.0013
0 + changes 0–10	10–25	0.996	0.993	0.0000

excess of all other causes of death. Altogether, a high rank position of the canonical variable V_i is obtained with low levels of cholesterol and decreases of cholesterol (or limited increases) plus low prevalence of smoking habits, whereas a high rank position of the canonical variable Ui is obtained with low levels of CHD and low levels of STR. Once more, the biologically coherent association is mainly that between population cholesterol level and CHD rates.

In order to test the stability of the canonical correlation, the solution for the 10-year mortality data was recomputed after having randomly excluded 2 of the 16 cohorts (Zutphen and Tanushimaru). The solution with the remaining 14 cohorts produced a canonical correlation of 0.946, which is exactly the same as that obtained with 16 cohorts. The estimated canonical variables V and U of the two excluded populations fit very well in the plot of the 14.

The canonical correlation was computed also using the mortality data of 5, 15, and 20 years of follow-up, although tabulated details are not provided here. However, a summary of all the canonical correlation analyses is given in Table 12. It appears that the best canonical correlation is obtained when the baseline levels of risk factors and their changes in 10 years are related to delayed mortality that occurred between year 10 and year 25 of follow-up.

Discussion

Analyses relating the mean levels of major CVD risk factors in the various population samples to the subsequent incidence or mortality rates can be found in classical monographs concerning the first 5- and 10-year follow-up periods of this study [2,4]. Usually they were limited to the CHD experience, since the Seven Countries Study focused on that problem and the measured risk factors were mainly cardiovascular risk factors. In more recent publications concerning longer follow-up periods [11–13], the same type of analysis confirmed the high correlation between mean levels of cholesterol and subsequent CHD mortality, although slightly less strong for longer follow-up periods. Similarly high correlations were found between entry levels of blood pressure and CHD mortality, which, however, were largely confounded by the association between blood pressure and cholesterol. However, the relationships between populations of the cholesterol/blood pressure product to CHD mortality in 10 years produced a high correlation coefficient ($r = 0.85$, against 0.82 with cholesterol alone and 0.71 with blood pressure alone).

In a publication covering the 20-year experience of 12 of the 16 cohorts, the inverse (ecologic) relationship between blood pressure and STR mortality was explained by the confounding effect of cholesterol level, whereas the individual relationship of blood pressure to STR mortality was always very high within cohorts [14]. In the present analysis, a more systematic approach was taken toward the relationship of mean risk factor levels to the mortality pattern, in the longest possible follow-up period of 25 years, making some comparisons with the 10-year experience as reference, and using also a rarely employed model (i.e., the canonical correlation analysis).

In general, the usual relationships were confirmed between mean levels of serum cholesterol and CHD mortality among the 16 cohorts. Moreover, in the canonical analysis the role of cholesterol changes was confirmed in the first 10 years of follow-up as predictors of CHD mortality in the subsequent 15 years [13,15].

The significant inverse relationship of cholesterol and blood pressure to STR mortality found in the univariate analysis (simple linear regression and correlation) was partly due to the high intercohort correlation of blood pressure to cholesterol. This means that populations having high cholesterol and high blood pressure levels suffer more from CHD than from STR. This may also mean that when cholesterol is not very high and blood pressure is only relatively high, other factors may intervene favoring the occurrence of STR. In addition, there is an inverse correlation between CHD and STR rates ($r = -0.42$ from Table 4) and a large direct ecologic correlation between serum cholesterol and the CHD/STR ratio ($r = 0.78$ in 10 years and 0.87 in 25 years). Moreover, in a partial correlation with the four factors kept fixed, the inverse correlation of CHD to STR rates becomes positive and of the same magnitude.

All of this leads to a hypothesis of competing risks, which is reinforced by a mean age at death that is 2.15 years higher among the STR deaths than among the CHD deaths when computed in the whole Seven Countries Study material. Finally, it should not be forgotten that the intercohort variability of blood pressure was small, and therefore a high association between blood pressure and death rates from STR could not be expected.

The high correlation between blood pressure and lung cancer and between cholesterol and lung cancer are likely a reflection of the association of blood pressure with smoking habits ($r = 0.38$) which may have obscured the expected relationship of smokers' prevalence to LUCA. However, positive relationships between high blood pressure and cancer have been found in other studies [16–18], as well as between dietary cholesterol and lung cancer [19].

From this point of view, the analysis of the force of cigarette smoking on disease and death among these population samples is likely disturbed by the different brands of cigarettes smoked in those years in the various countries. Turkish tobacco was popular in the Mediterranean countries, Virginia tobacco in the United States and the Netherlands, "Russian tobacco" was common in Finland, and several brands were used in Japan. When the 16 cohorts were ranked by smoking prevalence and by LUCA death rates, 10 of them fitted well with the expected relationship, 3 had relatively low cigarette consumption and high LUCA rates (U.S. railroad, West Finland, and Dalmatia), and 3 ranked high in smoking habits but low in LUCA death rates (Zrenjanin and the two Japanese cohorts). The possible different impact of Virginia versus Turkish tobacco may help to explain the apparently paradoxical experience of the U.S. railroad and of West Finland and Zrenjanin, but not of Dalmatia, whereas only some special protection can be claimed for the low LUCA rates in Japan. Other nonmeasured environmental factors could make the residual difference in explanation of the phenomena.

On the other hand, a distinct positive relationship of smokers' prevalence to OCA contrasts with the limited relationship of smokers' prevalence to LUCA. Finally, the effect of competing risks could have occurred between LUCA and chronic bronchitis because the rates of the latter were included in those of other causes of death (OTH).

In spite of the limited relationship of single factors to single causes of death, the multiple regression analysis was able, mainly in the 25-year data, to produce rather high r squared values and corresponding P values.

The canonical analysis was an attempt to obtain an overall view of the mortality picture as a function of the four chosen risk factors. The results were contrasting. Canonical analysis is one of the less commonly employed multivariate techniques whose limited use may be due, at least in part, to the difficulty in trying to interpret the results. In particular, it is traditionally rather easy to understand a linear combination of a number of possible independent variables, whereas it is much more difficult to understand a linear combination of dependent variables. Incidentally, using this set of data, it has been shown that the canonical variable U_i in 25 years has no correlation with the all-causes mortality ($r = 0.06$), indicating that, in the canonical variable U, death rates belonging to the several diagnostic groupings are not simply additive but are modeled by the weight of the coefficients, which keeps their relationship with the correspondent canonical variable V_i.

By this approach it became clear that high levels of blood pressure, cholesterol, and smoking habit did in fact correspond to high levels of death rates from CHD, LUCA, and OCA, all this contrasting with low levels of death rates from STR.

The overwhelming role of cholesterol, and of changes in cholesterol levels in relation to CHD death rates as shown by the solution of the canonical equation, which included the risk factor changes, likely reflects that CHD was the most common cause of death (among the various populations) and at the same time one with the largest variability and changes over time. The same applies to serum cholesterol which, on the side of possible causes, was the characteristic with the largest variability among cohorts and over time. Specific analyses on the role of changing cholesterol levels and changing CHD death rates were published elsewhere [13,15]. We mainly found increasing levels of serum cholesterol in the Serbian cohorts, paralleled by marked increases in CHD mortality rates, compared with all other cohorts and nations.

Although marginally, the relative increases in smokers' prevalence (or better, the relative changes in smokers' prevalence) were paralleled by high levels of LUCA.

In general, this comprehensive analysis tends to suggest that, whatever the analytical approach, the weight of mean cholesterol levels and the weight of CHD rates tend to condition the mortality patterns in these populations and their relationship with measured risk factors. This remains a major lesson from the long-term experience of the Seven Countries Study.

Acknowledgment. Research partly developed within the Italian National Research Council (CNR) targeted project "Prevention and Control of Disease Factors" (FATMA), subproject Community Medicine, Contract CNR93.0073.PF41.

References

1. Keys A, Aravanis C, Blackburn HW, van Buchem FSP, Buzina R, Djordjevic BS, Dontas AS, Fidanza F, Karvonen MJ, Kimura N, Lekos D, Monti M, Puddu V, Taylor HL (1967) Epidemiological studies related to coronary heart disease: characteristics of men aged 40–59 in seven countries. Acta Med Scand 460 [Suppl]180: 1–392
2. Keys A, Blackburn H, Menotti A, Buzina R, Mohacek I, Karvonen MJ, Punsar S, Aravanis C, Corcondilas A, Dontas AS, Lekos D, Fidanza F, Puddu V, Taylor HL, Monti M, Kimura N, van Buchem FSP, Djordjevic BS, Strasser T, Anderson JT, Den Hartog C, Pekkarinen M, Roine P, Sdrin H (1970) Coronary heart disease in seven countries. Circulation 41 [Suppl I]:1–211
3. Keys A, Aravanis C, Blackburn II, van Buchem FSP, Buzina R, Djordjevic BS, Fidanza F, Karvonen M, Menotti A, Puddu V, Taylor H (1972) Probability of middle-aged men developing coronary heart disease in five years. Circulation 45: 815–826
4. Keys A, Aravanis C, Blackburn H, Buzina R, Djordjevic BS, Dontas AS, Fidanza F, Karvonen MJ, Kimura N, Menotti A, Mohacek I, Nedeljkovic S, Puddu V, Punsar S, Taylor HL, van Buchem FSP (1980) Seven Countries Study. A multivariate analysis of death and coronary heart disease. Harvard University Press, Cambridge, Mass, London, pp 1–381
5. Keys A, Aravanis C, van Buchem F, Blackburn H, Buzina R, Djordjevic B, Fidanza F, Karvonen MJ, Kimura N, Menotti A, Nedeljkovic S, Puddu V, Taylor HL (1981) The diet and all causes death rate in the Seven Countries Study. Lancet 2:58–61

6. Menotti A, Capocaccia R, Conti S, Farchi G, Mariotti S, Verdecchia A, Keys A, Karvonen MJ, Punsar S (1977) Identifying subsets of major risk factors in multivariate estimation of coronary risk. J Chron Dis 30:557–565
7. Rose G, Blackburn H (1968) Manual on cardiovascular survey methods. World Health Organization, Geneva
8. Anderson JT, Keys A (1956) Cholesterol in serum and lipoprotein fractions: its measurements and stability. Clin Chem 2:145–159
9. World Health Organization (1965) International classification of diseases. 8th rev. World Health Organization, Geneva
10. Afifi AA, Clark V (1990) Computer-aided multivariate analysis. Van Norstrand Reinhold, New York, pp 1–505
11. Keys A, Menotti A, Aravanis C, Blackburn H, Djordjevic BS, Buzina R, Dontas A, Fidanza F, Karvonen MJ, Kimura N, Mohacek I, Nedeljkovic S, Puddu V, Punsar S, Taylor HL, Conti S, Kromhout D, Toshima H (1984) The Seven Countries Study: 2289 deaths in 15 years. Prev Med 13:141–154
12. Menotti A, Keys A, Aravanis C, Blackburn H, Dontas A, Fidanza F, Karvonen MJ, Kromhout D, Nedeljkovic S, Nissinen A, Pekkanen J, Punsar S, Seccareccia F, Toshima H (1989) Seven Countries Study. First 20 year mortality data in 12 cohorts of the Seven Countries. Ann Med 21:175–179
13. Menotti A, Keys A, Kromhout D, Blackburn H, Aravanis C, Bloemberg B, Buzina R, Dontas A, Fidanza F, Giampaoli S, Karvonen M, Lanti P, Mohacek I, Nedeljkovic S, Nissinen A, Pekkanen J, Punsar S, Seccareccia F, Toshima H (1993) Intercohort differences in coronary heart disease mortality in the 25-year follow-up of the Seven Countries Study. Eur J Epidemiol 9:527–536
14. Menotti A, Keys A, Blackburn H, Aravanis C, Dontas A, Fidanza F, Giampaoli S, Karvonen M, Kromhout D, Nedeljkovic S, Nissinen A, Pekkanen J, Punsar S, Seccareccia F, Toshima H (1990) Twenty-year stroke mortality and prediction in twelve cohorts of the Seven Countries Study. Int J Epidemiol 19:309–315
15. Menotti A (1993) Impact of international cardiovascular epidemiological studies on prevention: the Seven Countries Study. Can J Cardiol 9 [Suppl D]:8D–9D
16. Dyer AR, Stamler J, Berkson DM, Lindberg HA, Stevens E (1975) High blood pressure: a risk factor for cancer mortality? Lancet 1:1051–1056
17. Raynor WJ Jr, Shekelle RB, Rossof AH, Maliza C, Paul O (1981) High blood pressure and 17 year cancer mortality in the Western Electric Health Study. Am J Epidemiol 113:371–377
18. Khaw KT, Barrett-Connor E (1984) Systolic blood pressure and cancer mortality in an elderly population. Am J Epidemiol 120:550–558
19. Heilborn LK, Nomura AMY, Stemmermann GN (1984) Dietary cholesterol and lung cancer risk among Japanese men in Hawaii. Am J Clin Nutr 39:375–379

Discussion

R. Luepker: What does it add to or subtract from our interpretation of the Seven Countries Study by looking at a fewer number of units, that is, 7 versus 16 or 18 cohorts?

A. Menotti: Sometimes differences between cohorts *within* countries are relatively large, making for difficulties in pooling the data. That approach might be used, however, to look at regional death rates versus regional food consumption, telling more about differences in patterns rather than in single conditions. Of course, there are many limitations in that kind of analysis.

But whatever type of analysis used, the relationship between serum cholesterol and coronary heart disease remains throughout.

R. Beaglehole: Thank you very much for your fascinating presentation. Some of your data show that serum cholesterol level in the Japanese cohorts is declining, yet we have heard the last week about an increase in cholesterol mean values in Japanese national cross-sectional surveys. Is this difference due to cohort versus cross-sectional looks at data?

A. Menotti: These were two small Japanese units on the island of Kyushu, examined as cohorts and as separate cross-sections. They show small changes toward a decline in cholesterol levels. Perhaps our Japanese colleagues could provide more information on this point in regard to Tanishimaru and Ushibuka cohorts, or laboratory drift.

(Editor: Despite the lack of increase over time in serum cholesterol levels in the Kyushu cohorts in the Seven Countries Study, stroke rates have decreased. This may be a model, previously missing in Japan, suggesting that it is *not* the increase in serum cholesterol levels that is important in the reduced stroke deaths in Japan, but rather the decrease in blood pressure level.)

R. Luepker: I am impressed with the increased strength of associations when follow-up is extended out 15 to 25 years. This indicates that the measurements were well made to begin with, as well as their predictive power. Your findings about the changing cholesterol levels in Serbia and increased coronary disease rate are surely an important observation.

Dietary Saturated Fatty Acids, Serum Cholesterol, and Coronary Heart Disease

DAAN KROMHOUT and BENNIE P.M. BLOEMBERG

Summary. Different study designs show similar relations between serum cholesterol and coronary heart disease. On a cross-cultural level, average serum cholesterol levels and long-term mortality rates from coronary heart disease are strongly related in the Seven Countries Study. This association was also observed at the individual level. Within each cohort, the hazard ratio for coronary heart disease mortality increased 28% per mmol/l serum cholesterol level. However, the absolute risk level for coronary heart disease mortality differed much between cohorts, being lowest in the Japanese and Mediterranean cohorts and highest in the northern European and American cohorts.

The observed associations between dietary fatty acids and serum cholesterol first seem to be dependent on the study design. Average saturated fatty acid intake and average serum cholesterol level are strongly related in cross-cultural analysis (ecologic correlations) of the Seven Countries Study data. However, Within the Zutphen Study and several other cohorts, zero or low-order correlations were observed between individual intake of saturated fatty acids and serum cholesterol level. In contrast, strong associations have been observed between changes in saturated fatty acid intake and changes in serum cholesterol in controlled experiments. This difference may largely be due to measurement error. For example, when in the Zutphen Study, instead of a single dietary fatty acid intake assessment, five repeated measures were used, significant associations were found between dietary saturated fatty acid intake and serum cholesterol.

It may be concluded that the observed relation between serum cholesterol and coronary heart disease mortality is independent of the study design. Dietary saturated fatty acids are related to serum cholesterol at the population but not at the individual level. If, however, measurement error is taken into account, associations are also observed between dietary saturated fatty acids and serum cholesterol at the individual level.

Key words. Dietary saturated fatty acids—Serum cholesterol—Coronary heart disease

Introduction

The so-called diet–cholesterol hypothesis of the cause of coronary heart disease has been studied from an epidemiological point of view since the beginning of this century. The Dutch internist De Langen found low cholesterol levels in the inhabitants of the island of Java, Indonesia, compared with the Dutch [1]. He suggested that hypercholesterolemia was associated with metabolic diseases (e.g., diabetes and atherosclerotic complications). He also did an experiment in two patients showing an increase in serum cholesterol on a diet high in eggs, meat, and milk. In Snapper's famous book, *Chinese Lessons to Western Medicine*, published in 1941, atherosclerotic complications were reportedly almost nonexistent in northern China while the incidence of these diseases was increasing in the United States and Europe [2]. Snapper suggested that these differences are not due to genetics but that differences in nutrition of the Chinese and the Westerners give a better explanation. He stated,

The Chinese diet contains only small amounts of cholesterol but considerable quantities of unsaturated acids especially of linoleic and linolenic acid. It is certain that the average cholesterol content of the blood of the Chinese is lower than that of the Westerners and this gives perhaps an indication why the tendency of lipoid infiltration of the vessel wall is so much smaller among the Chinese.

These examples show that already in the first half of this century, evidence was presented for the so-called diet–cholesterol hypothesis based on cross-cultural comparisons.

It took until the 1950s, however, before systematic epidemiologic studies investigating the hypothesis took place. Keys and coworkers showed that mortality from coronary heart disease was high in the United States and Finland but low in the Mediterranean countries of Italy and Spain [3]. The countries with high mortality rates from coronary heart disease were characterized by high serum cholesterol levels and a high fat intake. These early observations formed the basis for the Seven Countries Study that started in 1958. Seven Countries data will be used to describe the relations between serum cholesterol and coronary heart disease and those between serum cholesterol and dietary saturated fatty acids. Special attention will be paid to measurement error in cross-sectional dietary surveys.

The Seven Countries Study

Between 1958 and 1964, 12 763 men aged 40 to 59 from 16 different cohorts were enrolled in the Seven Countries Study. Eleven cohorts consisted of men living in rural parts of Finland, Italy, Greece, former Yugoslavia, and Japan. The other five were two cohorts of railroad employees (United States, Italy), one of workers in a large cooperative in Zrenjanin (Serbia), one of university professors in Belgrade, and one of inhabitants of Zutphen, a small commercial town in the Netherlands. The characteristics of these cohorts have been described in detail previously [4–6].

In most of these 16 cohorts, medical examinations were carried out at baseline and after 5 and 10 years of follow-up [4–6]. Standardized medical questionnaires were filled out [4], a physical examination made, and electrocardiograms and blood pressure, height, and weight were measured in a standardized way. Venous blood samples were taken and serum cholesterol was measured in a standardized way in a central laboratory.

The vital status of all men was checked at regular intervals and completed after 25 years for all 16 cohorts. Information about the underlying cause of death was collected from general practitioners and local hospitals, and copies of death certificates obtained. The final coding of the underlying cause of death was done at the coordination center during the first 10 years of follow-up by H. Blackburn and A. Menotti in Minneapolis, USA and between 10 and 25 years of follow-up by A. Menotti in Rome. Almost 6000 men (47%) died during 25 years of follow-up. The serum cholesterol and coronary heart disease mortality data were used to study the associations between these variables at both the population and the individual level.

Dietary information was collected at baseline in small random samples (8–49 men) of each cohort using the dietary record method [7]. Food tables with detailed information on the fatty acid composition of foods in the Seven Countries were lacking in the 1960s. Therefore, the fatty acid composition of duplicate portions was determined for 13 of the 16 cohorts and analyses were carried out at the Laboratory of Physiological Hygiene, University of Minnesota, Minneapolis, USA. These data were used to relate the average saturated fatty acid intake of the different cohorts at baseline with the 5- and 10-year occurrence of coronary heart disease [5,6].

Later the investigators became interested in the effect of individual fatty acids on serum cholesterol. They also became interested in the effect of other nutrients, nonnutrients, and foods on the occurrence of chronic diseases. Therefore, the original dietary intake data were recoded in a standardized way by one dietitian in 1985 and 1986. The average food intake of men in the 16 cohorts was summarized in 16 food groups [7]. In 1987, foods representing the baseline diet were bought locally and sent by air in cooling boxes to the Netherlands. Within 1 day after arrival, foods were washed, cleaned, and combined into food composites in the laboratory of the Department of Human Nutrition, Agricultural University, Wageningen, (head: M.B. Katan), representing the average food intake of each cohort. Food composites were subsequently homogenized and stored at −20°C until analyses took place. The individual fatty acid content of each of the 16 food composites was determined (D. Kromhout et al., manuscript in preparation), and the data used to study associations between individual saturated fatty acids and serum cholesterol, at the population or cohort level.

All men in Zutphen (the Netherlands) were surveyed with the dietary history method in 1960, 1965, 1970, 1985, and 1990. This method was also used in

Crevalcore (Italy) in 1965, 1970, and 1991, and in Montegiorgio (Italy) in 1965 and 1991. In 1969, a dietary survey using the dietary history method was also carried out in East and West Finland, and repeated 20 years later in 1989. Recently, the dietary data collected between 1960 and 1970 in the Netherlands, Italy, and Finland were coded in a standardized way. In total, 16 main food groups were established and computerized food tables containing the foods used in the 1960s and their nutrient content were prepared for the three countries. These data were then used to study associations between intake of saturated fatty acids and serum cholesterol on an individual level in three European cultures. Five dietary surveys were carried out in Zutphen between 1960 and 1990 and these data were used to study the effect of measurement error on the association between dietary saturated fatty acids and serum cholesterol in individuals within cohorts.

Serum Cholesterol and Coronary Heart Disease Mortality

Analysis at the population level showed that average serum cholesterol level was strongly related to 5-year incidence of and mortality from coronary heart disease [5]. Similar results were found using the 10-year coronary heart disease mortality data [6]. Thus, coronary heart disease mortality rates are high in cultures with high average serum cholesterol levels (e.g., Finland and the United States) and low in cultures with relatively low average serum cholesterol levels (e.g., Greece and Japan).

Analyses at the individual level showed that serum cholesterol is an important predictor of coronary heart disease incidence and mortality after 5 and 10 years of follow-up [5,6]. However, the predictive value is quite different in different cultures. Strong associations were observed in the United States and northern Europe [5,6], while associations were much weaker in southern Europe and Japan. Therefore, in recent analyses, serum cholesterol was related to long-term coronary heart disease mortality in seven "homogeneous groups." Due to small numbers in most of the cohorts, the cohorts were regrouped based on cultural resemblance and dynamics of serum cholesterol levels during the first 10 years of follow-up. These analyses showed that 25-year mortality from coronary heart disease varied between 5% in Greece and 30% in East Finland. In each group the hazard ratio for coronary heart disease mortality increased 28% per mmol/l increase in serum cholesterol. However, the absolute risk level for coronary heart disease mortality differed much between cohorts, being lowest in the Japanese and Mediterranean cohorts and highest in the northern European and American cohorts. At a serum cholesterol level of 5 mmol/l, the 25-year mortality rate from coronary heart disease varied between about 2.5% in the Japanese and Mediterranean cohorts and greater than 10% in the northern European and American cohorts. Serum cholesterol level is therefore a strong predictor in every culture, but the absolute level of risk may vary depending on the presence of other risk factors for coronary heart disease.

Large-scale intervention studies have shown that a decrease in serum cholesterol leads to a decrease in coronary heart disease incidence and mortality. A recent meta-analysis of a number of intervention trials showed that a decrease in serum cholesterol of 1% is associated with a decrease in coronary heart disease mortality of at least 2% [8]. It may therefore be concluded that results from observational and experimental epidemiological studies have shown that serum cholesterol is an important determinant of coronary heart disease risk. However, the absolute coronary heart disease risk of elevated serum cholesterol is strongly dependent on the culture.

Dietary Saturated Fatty Acids and Serum Cholesterol

In ecological analysis, the average intake of saturated fatty acids of the Seven Countries cohorts was strongly related to the average serum cholesterol level [5]. When the results of the recent fatty acid analyses were used, the strongest association was found for saturated fatty acids with 12 and 14 carbon atoms, lauric and myristic acid (D. Kromhout et al., manuscript in preparation). These results are consistent with those of dietary interventions in which saturated fatty acids with 12, 14, and 16 atoms (e.g., lauric, myristic, and palmitic acid) have the strongest serum cholesterol elevating effect.

In the Zutphen Study, however, and in several other cohort studies, zero or low-order correlations were found between the intake of saturated fat and serum cholesterol in individuals, using cross-sectional data [9–12]. In contrast, strong effects were observed consistently in controlled experiments. In a recently published meta-analysis of 27 controlled experiments, it was shown that a change of 1% of energy in saturated fatty acids (with 12–16 carbon atoms) was associated with a change of 0.056 mmol/l (2.2 mg/dl) in serum cholesterol [13]. This is similar to the effect predicted from the Keys equation developed in the 1960s [14]. This difference between the results on the individual level, in cohort studies using cross-sectional data, and those of controlled experiments, may be due to measurement error in the epidemiological studies.

Already in 1965, Keys discussed the influence of measurement error on the relationship between fatty acid intake and serum cholesterol [15]. Later, Jacobs and coworkers described the statistical background of low-order correlations between fatty acids and serum cholesterol in observational studies on individuals [16]. Liu and coworkers discussed the influence on this relationship of measurement error in the food record method [17]. In all of these papers the random (intraindividual) error in measurement was discussed. However, in the dietary history method used in the Zutphen Study and in several other cohort studies, interindividual error also plays an important role. The effect of these errors could be investigated in the Zutphen Study because information on diet and serum cholesterol was collected repeatedly. By analyzing changes in dietary intake, the interindividual error can be accounted for.

Five measurements on diet and serum cholesterol were collected in the Zutphen Study between 1960 and 1990. To exclude the between-person variation in serum cholesterol, changes in fatty acid intake were related to changes in serum cholesterol (B.P.M. Bloemberg and D. Kromhout, manuscript in preparation). The results of these analyses showed that the relation between dietary fatty acids and serum cholesterol was on average stronger when changes were considered instead of levels. The interindividual error may play a smaller role when changes in dietary intake are considered. Due to the intraindividual error in the measurement of fatty acids intake, the regression coefficient for changes in saturated fatty acids on changes in serum cholesterol was 30% lower than the one found in controlled experiments.

It can be concluded that saturated fatty acid intake is strongly related to serum cholesterol level and its change. Measurement error attenuates this relation to a large extent when studied on the individual level using cross-sectional data.

Conclusions

The observed relation between serum cholesterol level and coronary heart disease is independent of the study design. Strong associations are described in descriptive, cohort, and experimental studies. Saturated fatty acids are strongly related to serum cholesterol in descriptive and intervention studies. No association is found in analyses on the individual level using cross-sectional data. If, however, measurement error is taken into account properly (e.g., by using repeatedly collected data), associations are found between changes in dietary saturated fatty acids and changes in serum cholesterol at the individual level. It is concluded that overwhelming evidence indicates that serum cholesterol level is an important determinant of coronary heart disease mortality and that saturated fatty acids are a major influence on serum cholesterol levels, for individuals and for populations.

References

1. Langen CD de (1916) Cholesterol metabolism and racial pathology (in Dutch). Geneesk T Ned Indie 56:1–34
2. Snapper I (1941) Chinese lessons to Western medicine. Interscience, New York, p. 158
3. Keys A (1983) From Naples to seven countries. A sentimental journey. Prog Biochem Pharmacol 19:1–30
4. Keys A, Aravanis C, Blackburn HW, van Buchem FSP, Buzina R, Djordjevic BS, Dontas AS, Fidanza F, Karvonen MJ, Kimura N, Lekos D, Monti M, Puddu V, Taylor HL (1967) Epidemiological studies related to coronary heart disease: characteristics of men aged 40–59 in seven countries. Acta Med Scand 460[Suppl 180]:1–392
5. Keys A (1970) Coronary heart disease in seven countries. Circulation 41[Suppl I]:1–211

6. Keys A (1980) Seven Countries. A multivariate analysis of death and coronary heart disease. Harvard University Press, Cambridge, Mass., pp 1–381

7. Kromhout D, Keys A, Aravanis C, Buzina R, Fidanza F, Giampaoli S, Jansen A, Menotti A, Nedeljkovic S, Pekkarinen M, Simic BS, Toshima H (1989) Food consumption patterns in the 1960s in seven countries. Am J Clin Nutr 49:889–894

8. Holme I (1990) An analysis of randomized trials evaluating the effect of cholesterol reduction on total mortality and coronary heart disease incidence. Circulation 98:206–210

9. Kromhout D (1983) Body weight, diet and serum cholesterol in 871 middle-aged men during 10 years of follow-up (the Zutphen Study). Am J Clin Nutr 38:591–598

10. Kannel WB, Gordon T (eds) (1970) The Framingham Study: An epidemiological investigation of cardiovascular disease. Section 24: The Framingham Diet Study: Diet and the regulation of serum cholesterol. U.S. Government Printing Office, Washington, D.C.

11. Nichols AB, Ravenscroft C, Lamphiear DE, Ostrander LD Jr (1976) Independence of serum lipid levels and dietary habits. The Tecumseh Study. J Am Med Ass 236:1948–1963

12. Shekelle RB, Shryock AM, Paul O, Lepper M, Stamler J, Liu S, Raynor WJ (1981) Diet, serum cholesterol, and death from coronary heart disease. The Western Electric Study. N Engl J Med 304:65–70

13. Mensink RP, Katan MB (1992) Effect of dietary fatty acids on serum lipids and lipoproteins. A meta-analysis of 27 trials. Arterioscler Thromb 12:911–919

14. Keys A, Anderson JT, Grande F (1965) Serum cholesterol response to changes in diet. IV. Particular saturated fatty acids in the diet. Metabolism 14:776–787

15. Keys A (1965) Dietary survey methods in studies on cardiovascular epidemiology. Voeding 26:464–483

16. Jacobs DR, Anderson JT, Blackburn H (1979) Diet and serum cholesterol: do zero correlations negate the relationship? Am J Epidemiol 110:77–87

17. Liu K, Stamler J, Dyer A, McKeever J, McKeever P (1978) Statistical methods to assess and minimize the role of intra-individual variability in observing the relationship between dietary lipids and serum cholesterol. J Chron Dis 31:399–418

Discussion

R. Luepker: Would you elaborate, Dr. Kromhout, on your findings about the relationship between absolute intake of C:12, C:14 chain length fatty acids and serum cholesterol level, compared to the percent fat calorie intake from those fatty acids? Is that adjusted for total fat intake?

D. Kromhout: We expressed the intake of fatty acids as percent of dietary calories, adjusting for total caloric intake. We did *not* adjust for total fat intake but adjusted for energy intake. The association between total energy intake and serum cholesterol level is small, so that using absolute amounts in grams of fatty acids, the relationship to serum cholesterol level is quite similar to percent calories.

Functional Capacity in 70- to 89-year-old Men in Finland, Italy, and the Netherlands

Aulikki Nissinen, Paula Kivinen, Edith Feskens,
Simona Giampaoli, Daan Kromhout, Alessandro Menotti,
Sirkka-Liisa Kivelä, and Martti Karvonen

Summary. Functional and mental capacities were studied in the 30-year follow-up survey of the Finnish, Italian, and Dutch cohorts of the Seven Countries Study. The aim was to find lifestyle-related factors in middle age which predict functional capacity in old age. This analysis focuses on the variation between cohorts in different cultural settings and with different histories of coronary heart disease and risk factors. In 1989–1991, 1411 men performed the standard examination and tests on activities of daily living (ADL); mental, psychic and physical functioning; and self-perceived health.

Functional capacity (ADL) was good, ranging 65%–72% in the Finnish men, 63%–78% in the Italians, and 84% in Dutch men ($P < 0.001$). Mental functioning measured by the mean values of the Mini-Mental State Examination (MMSE) was 23.8–24.5 in Finland, 23.1–23.3 in Italy, and 26.2 in the Netherlands ($P < 0.001$). The results indicate that men in Finland and Italy had lower capacity in ADL and mental functioning compared with their counterparts in the Netherlands.

Great variation was observed in self-perceived health. Only 10%–22% of men in Finland reported feeling healthy or very healthy, compared to 72%–86% in Italy and 89% in the Netherlands ($P < 0.001$).

These results show great variation between the different cohorts. In general, functional capacity was best among Dutch men and poorest among men in East Finland.

Key words. Self-rated health—Physical capacity—Functional capacity—Physical performance—Elderly

Introduction

Functional capacity is a multidimensional concept that includes physical, psychological, and social components and is closely related to life circumstances. In old age, good functional capacity means a high degree of independence, quality of life, and well-being, regardless of (diagnosed) current diseases [1,2].

The Seven Countries Study started in the late 1950s to examine how lifestyle-related factors such as smoking and diet, biological risk factors (e.g., serum cholesterol and blood pressure) explain the onset of coronary heart disease among middle-aged men [3,4]. The 30-year follow-up survey has been conducted in three European countries, Finland, Italy, and the Netherlands, among men in cohorts 70 to 89 years old at the time of the survey (1989–1991).

Elaboration of coronary heart disease determinants was the original aim of the Seven Countries Study. As the men became older, another focus of the follow-up survey was to assess their capacity for daily life and, in the broadest sense, autonomy in old age. The ultimate goal is to identify lifestyle-related factors in middle age which predict functional capacity in the elderly. This article presents information on functional capacity of cohorts of elderly men in different cultural settings.

Materials and Methods

At the time of the 30-year follow-up in 1989–1991, 205 men from eastern (East) and 265 from southwestern (West) Finland, 238 men from Crevalcore (Italy) and 191 from Montegiorgio (Italy), and 560 men from Zutphen (The Netherlands) participated in the survey. Participation rates were 88% in East and 91% in West Finland, 57% in Crevalcore, 58% in Montegiorgio, and 78% in Zutphen. Men living in institutions were excluded from the analyses.

A common protocol used in the previous surveys [4] was completed with new aspects of geriatric interest collected in a standardized way in the three countries [5,6]. The survey included questionnaires, clinical examination, physical performance measurements, and mental and psychic status examination. Invitations to the examination were mailed about 2 weeks prior to the study. Questionnaires concerning socioeconomic status, health behavior and other health-related issues, symptoms, activities of daily living, other physical activities, hobbies, and social relations were filled in by the subjects at home and returned at the examination center. The questionnaires were checked by technicians for missing or inconsistent answers and completed accordingly.

Mental capacity was examined with the Mini-Mental State Examination (MMSE) [7]. Firstly the MMSE was done and participants scoring a total of 27 points or less were then tested using a clinical dementia rating test [8].

The questionnaire contained a list of 14 tasks. Questions concerning ability to prepare meals and do heavy domestic tasks (e.g., to wash windows and floors) were excluded from the analysis as being irrelevant for elderly men. We used 12 items to construct two indexes of functional capacity, and measured basic activities of daily living (BADL) and functional mobility in specific physical activities (MOB).

BADL consisted of the following activities: walking between rooms, going to the toilet, washing and bathing, dressing and undressing, going to bed and getting up, and eating.

MOB consisted of the following activities: going outdoors, negotiating stairs, walking at least 400 m, carrying heavy weights, cutting toenails, and doing light domestic tasks.

The answers to each item of the questionnaire were classified into four categories: (1) Not able to manage the function. (2) Needs help to manage the function. (3) Able to manage the function with some difficulty. (4) Able to manage the function without difficulty. For constructing a functional capacity index, categories 1 and 2 were recorded to 0. Thus, for both indexes a total of 24 points means an ability to perform activities without help and without difficulties, a sum of 18–23 means ability to perform activities without help but with some difficulties, and a sum below 17 means one or more limited activities.

A functional capacity index was then composed from BADL and MOB indexes:

Good: BADL sum 24 plus MOB sum 18–24 points
Moderate: BADL sum 18–23 plus MOB sum 18–23 points, or
            BADL sum 24 plus MOB sum 0–17 points
Poor: BADL sum 0–17 points

The participants were requested to judge their health by four categories: very healthy, healthy, moderately healthy, not healthy. For analysis the categories "very healthy" and "healthy" were combined to a three-class self-rated health index: good, moderate, poor.

Physical performance tests were conducted by trained research assistants. The methods were the same as those used in the Established Populations for Epidemiologic Studies of the Elderly (EPESE) study, and training was conducted with EPESE's videotape [9]. These performance measurements included the timing of a 3-m gait course (the mean of two measurements was used in analyses), repeated chair stands (time required to stand up from an armless chair and sit down in the chair five times). Grip strength was measured with a sphygmomanometer twice for the dominant limb, and the mean value of these measurements was used in the analyses.

Analyses were performed with SAS statistical software [10]. Differences between areas in categorical variables were tested using analysis of maximum likelihood (Catmod procedure) and for continuous variables using a general linear model procedure. Cronbach's alfa reliability coefficient was used to test internal reliability of the constructed index of functional capacity. The effect of age was taken into account by using a direct age standardization, with the total population as reference.

Results

There were no remarkable differences between the cohorts in marital status. In Finland 73% of men in the east and 68% in the west were married compared to 72%–73% in Italy and 78% in the Netherlands. However, living status was

Table 1. Functional capacity (activities of daily living) in 70- to 89-year-old men in Finland, Italy, and the Netherlands, 1989–1991.

| | ADL-capacity class | | |
Cohort	Good (%)	Moderate (%)	Poor (%)
Finland			
East	65	29	6
West	72	19	9
Italy			
Montegiorgio	63	24	13
Crevalcore	78	13	9
The Netherlands			
Zutphen	84	14	3

Catmod procedure: age $P < 0.001$; area $P < 0.001$; age area $P =$ ns.
ADL, activities of daily living.

quite different between the three countries. Most men in Italy lived with their family (85%–92%) whereas only 72%–74% of men in Finland and 79% in the Netherlands had family with them. In East Finland 7% of mem were institutionalized and 20% lived alone. Among the other cohorts, 1%–4% were long-term hospitalized. In West Finland 25% of men lived alone; 17% lived alone in the Netherlands and only 11% in Italy.

Functional capacity was best among Dutch men and poorest among men in East Finland (Table 1). The proportion of those with good functional capacity (ADL) varied between 65%–72% among Finnish, 63%–78% among Italian, and 84% among the Dutch men ($P < 0.001$). The average time needed for five repeated chair stands was shortest among men in West Finland, 13.7 s and longest among men in Montegiorgio, Italy, 17.3 s (Table 2). Men in Zutphen, the Netherlands, were fastest in walking 3 ms, with an average of 3.1 s; men in West Finland were the slowest with 4.2 s. Grip strength was also weakest in West Finland, only 62.4 kPa compared with the strongest average value of 80.6 kPa among the men in Crevalcore, Italy.

Mental functioning described by the mean values of the MMSE was 23.8–24.5 in Finland, 23.1–23.3 in Italy, and 26.2 in the Netherlands ($P < 0.001$, Table 3). The men in East Finland and Italy had lower capacity in mental and in ADL functions than men in the Netherlands.

Wide variation was observed in self-perceived health (Table 4). Only 10%–22% of men in Finland reported feeling healthy or very healthy compared with 72%–86% in Italy and 89% in the Netherlands ($P < 0.001$).

Table 2. Physical function in 70- to 89-year-old men in Finland, Italy, and the Netherlands, 1989–1991.

Function and Cohort	No.	Mean	S.D.	Age-adjusted mean
Walking time (s)				
Finland				
East	182	3.8	1.7	3.8
West	237	4.2	1.6	4.1
Italy				
Montegiorgio	171	3.8	1.1	3.8
Crevalcore	216	3.7	2.3	3.6
The Netherlands				
Zutphen	526	3.1	0.9	3.0

GLM procedure: age $P < 0.001$; area $P < 0.001$; age area $P = $ ns.

	No.	Mean	S.D.	Age-adjusted mean
Repeated chair stand (s)				
Finland				
East	159	16.2	4.5	16.2
West	200	13.7	4.5	13.6
Italy				
Montegiorgio	153	17.3	3.6	17.3
Crevalcore	193	16.3	3.9	16.2
The Netherlands				
Zutphen	505	15.3	3.6	15.4

GLM procedure: age $P < 0.001$; area $P < 0.001$; age area $P = $ ns.

	No.	Mean	S.D.	Age-adjusted mean
Grip strength (kPa)				
Finland				
East	183	63.8	18.1	63.7
West	239	62.4	16.5	63.5
Italy				
Montegiorgio	172	70.5	20.7	69.8
Crevalcore	216	80.6	21.2	81.2
The Netherlands				
Zutphen	528	73.8	18.6	73.1

GLM procedure: age $P < 0.001$; area $P < 0.001$; age area $P = $ ns.

S.D., standard deviation.

Table 3. Mini-mental state examination (MMSE) in 70- to 89-year-old men in Finland, Italy, and the Netherlands, 1989–1991.

Cohort	No.	Mean	S.D.	Age-adjusted mean
Finland				
East	185	23.8	3.6	23.8
West	244	24.5	4.2	25.0
Italy				
Montegiorgio	192	23.3	5.5	23.2
Crevalcore	228	23.1	4.5	23.3
The Netherlands				
Zutphen	505	26.2	2.9	26.1

S.D., standard deviation.
GLM procedure: age $P < 0.001$; area $P < 0.001$; age area $P < 0.001$.

Table 4. Self-rated health in 70- to 89-year-old men in Finland, Italy, and the Netherlands, 1989–1991.

Cohort	Self-rated health (%)		
	Healthy or very healthy	Moderately healthy	Not healthy
Finland			
East	10	48	43
West	22	47	32
Italy			
Montegiorgio	72	22	5
Crevalcore	86	10	4
The Netherlands			
Zutphen	89	10	2

Catmod procedure: age P = ns; area $P < 0.001$; age area P = ns.

Discussion

The measurement of functional capacity in population studies is usually based on questionnaires; standardized performance tests are rarely used [11–14]. Though self-imposed assessments have limitations [15–17], they are widely used due to their feasibility. Standardized tests provide greater reproducibility and in some situations make it possible to obtain more reliable data on physical functioning [18]. They provide, however, limited information on how a person manages in his or her own environment [19].

In this survey we used both self-administered questionnaires and standard tests for the assessment of functional capacity. However, methodological short-comings remain, and the comparison between cohorts is hampered. A higher level of standardization was obtained for tests which measured physical capacity, such as walking time, repeated chair stand, and grip strength. Men in Zutphen, the Netherlands, performed well in these tests; men in East Finland had the poorest values. Differences within the same country are interesting: neither in Finland nor in Italy are the regional cohorts similar. Men in West Finland performed better than those in East Finland. These observations are in line with previous findings on cardiovascular morbidity, mortality, and risk factors in middle age [4,20].

The Mini-Mental State Examination is an internationally used questionnaire. Men in the Netherlands and West Finland had better mental function than their counterparts in the other cohorts. Performance in MMSE, probably is influenced by demographic factors (e.g., education), was higher in the Netherlands than in the other countries.

A self-administered questionnaire was used for the assessment of daily living and self-perceived health. The results varied surprisingly between the cohorts. Finnish men reported a lower capacity in activities of daily living and rated themselves less healthy than men in Italy and Holland. Cultural variation can underlie this observation. However, the prior history of morbidity and mortality from coronary heart disease, and their risk factors [4], support the view that men in Finland are less healthy and more dependent than men in Italy and in the Netherlands.

Acknowledgments. We thank the Academy of Science of Finland; the Medical Research Council, Finland; and the National Institute on Aging, United States (grant number EDC-1 1R01 AG08762-01A1) for financial support of the study. We are grateful for MSc Veli Koistinen for his assistance in statistical analyses.

References

1. Kuriansky JB, Gurland B, Fleiss J (1976) The assessment of self-care capacity in geriatric psychiatric patients by objective and subjective methods. J Clin Psychol 32:95–102
2. World Health Organization (1984) The uses of epidemiology in the study of the elderly. Technical Report Series #706, WHO, Geneva
3. Keys A (1953) Prediction and possible prevention of coronary heart disease. Am J Publ Health 43:1399–1407
4. Keys A (1970) Coronary heart disease in seven countries. Am Heart Assoc Monograph No 29, New York
5. Nissinen A, Tervahauta M, Pekkanen J, Kivinen P, Stengard J, Kaarsalo E, Kivela SL, Vaisanen S, Salonen JT, Tuomilehto J (1993) Cardiovascular risk factors among 70–89 year old Finnish men. Age Ageing 22:365–376
6. Lammi UK (1989) Functional capacity and associated factors in elderly Finnish men. Scand J Soc Med 17(1):67–75
7. Folstein MF, Folstein SE (1975) "Mini-Mental State." A practical method for grading the cognitive state of patients for the clinician. J Psychiatr Res 12:189
8. Hughes CP, Berg L, Danziger WL, Coben LA, Martin RL (1982) A new clinical scale for the staging of dementia. Br J Psychiat 140:566–572
9. "Assessing physical performance in the home." Training videotape
10. SAS Institute (1985) SAS user's guide: Statistics. SAS Institute, Cary, N.C.
11. Kuriansky J, Gurland B (1976) The performance test of activities of daily living. Int J Aging Human Devel 7:343–352
12. Jette AM, Branch LG (1984) Musculoskeletal impairment among the non-institutionalized aged. Int Rehabil Med 6:157–161
13. Jette AB, Branch LG (1985) Impairment and disability in the aged. J Chron Dis 38:59–65
14. Williams ME, Hornberger JC (1984) A quantitative method of identifying older persons at risk for increasing long term care services. J Chron Dis 37:705–711
15. Linn MW, Hynter KI, Linn BS (1980) Self-assessed health, impairment and disability in Anglo, Black and Cuban elderly. Med Care 18:282–288
16. Branch LG, Meyers AP (1987) Assessing physical function in the elderly. Clin Geriatr Med 3:29–51
17. Rowe JW, Kahn RL (1987) Human aging. Usual and successful. Science 237:143–149

18. Guyatt G, Walter S, Norman G (1987) Measuring change over time: assessing the usefulness of evaluative instruments. J Chron Dis 40:171–178
19. Tinetti ME, Ginter SF (1988) Identifying mobility dysfunctions in elderly patients. Standard neuromuscular examination or direct assessment? J Am Med Assoc 259:1190–1193
20. Menotti A, Keys A, Kromhout D, Nissinen A, Blackburn H, Fidanza F, Giampaoli S, Karvonen M, Pekkanen J, Punsar S, Seccreccia F (1991) All-cause mortality and its determinants in middle aged men in Finland, the Netherlands, and Italy in a 25 year follow up. J Epidemiol Commun Health 45:125–130

Discussion

Asian-Pacific Seminar student: Can you describe the proportion of individuals surviving the 30-year follow-up and, if there is a relationship, describe the correlation between functional capacity and survival in those still living?

A. Nissinen: Is the question whether functional capacity is related to survival because a large proportion of the participants may have died? We now have full data on Finland, The Netherlands, and Italy, with 30-year follow-up, and don't have all the answers. The basic question is very important, however: how the characteristics of lifestyle in middle age predict long-term survival and personal autonomy in old age. We just don't have the analyses completed yet.

D. Jacobs: Findings of self-perceived health status were remarkably different between these population groups. Do you have any information why there should be such a huge difference between Finns and the other populations?

A. Nissinen: We have subjective points of view about these men, but one of our problems is that institutionalized Finnish men were included in the survey. We must do analyses excluding institutionalized participants who have the weakest functional capacity. There seem to be real differences as well.

Professor Karvonen, who has followed men of similar age in Italy and Finland, would perhaps like to comment.

M. Karvonen: My subjective impression comes from visiting a good many of these men at their homes when they were not able to come to the survey center (a survey function which befits an elderly scientist in the field!). In many cases, I made examinations at home (capacities of the examiner and the participants may both have been bad!). But definitely, I met more people, more old men, laid up for health in the east of Finland than in the west. My fellow inhabitants in the fishing village of Pioppi, Italy, are in rather good shape. My hunch is that men of Pioppi in southern Italy are in better shape than their co-equals in east Finland, but I have made no age-specific analysis.

A. Nissinen: Most of these men of eastern Finland have atherosclerosis, coronary heart disease, and angina pectoris, real disease that affects their daily living and prevents them from saying that they are healthy.

R. Bonita: Would you comment on your findings of good self-rated health and daily activities and mental status among the Dutch men, who are nevertheless more often depressed?

A. Nissinen: It is true that our analysis shows that Dutch men are more often depressed than others, but we had to discard a great deal of data when all the questions were not answered. We have to explore this further in regard to biased response.

S. Hatano: Thank you for all this interesting information and the many possible hypotheses involved. We should recognize that the Seven Countries population is aging and the group provides an important cohort for further follow-up. It is quite ambitious that you have followed a small number of cohorts for 30 years. In my opinion, this is just wishful thinking because half the population will disappear in 10 more years time, many of them institutionalized, escaping objective survey methodology.

I say this because we have very long-term experience in studying old people in the Tokyo Gerontological Institute. The investigators have developed more subtle indicators of the quality of life, not only physical ability items, but those on social relationships and intellectual interests.

A. Nissinen: Thank you very much for your comment. We also have other measures of this difficult issue: quality of life. In respect to the small number remaining in the cohort, in any case, men do, indeed, die, so if we consider that the men represent eastern and western Finnish male populations, we can compare these results with other surveys of similar age in our country. The beauty of this study is its 35-year history and we don't necessarily need large numbers. We are quite aware of the analytical problems among survivors.

Food Intake Assessment for Epidemiological Studies

Flaminio Fidanza and Adalberta Alberti Fidanza

Summary. The dietary survey methods used in the European cohorts of the Seven Countries Study are described. Improved dietary history and food frequency methods are also described in more detail, including assessment of their validity. In large-scale surveys, a camera method and a videotel system are very promising. Because the correlation between vitamin and mineral intake and nutritional status assessed biochemically was not high, biochemical or functional methods to assess nutriture are highly recommended. In rapidly changing societies, the longitudinal assessment of food intake is compulsory.

Key words. Dietary survey methods—History—Weighed record—Camera Videotel

During the 30 years since the Seven Countries Study was initiated, its findings and those of many other studies have shown that dietary habits play a central role in the etiology of cardiovascular, neoplastic and other chronic diseases afflicting contemporary populations on a mass scale. Therefore, the information development and evaluation of food intake assessment methods for population studies have been—and continue to be—of great importance.

Weighed Record Method

In the Seven Countries Study, among the various methods for food consumption appraisal for European cohorts, the weighed record method was preferred. This is very likely because of previous experience with this method both at the Laboratory of Physiological Hygiene in Minneapolis (for the business and professional men participating in the long-term study of aging) and at the Department of Nutritional Chemistry in Helsinki (for studies on food consumption of rural families in East and West Finland).

Because this method is time-consuming and costly, a subsample of the cohort was selected with an original procedure. From the roster, half of the subsample subjects were selected at random, and the other half their closest neighbours.

In this way one dietitian could carry out the survey on two subjects at the same time [1].

In order to validate the food composition tables and assess fatty acid intake, it was necessary to carry out a chemical analysis of food composites or equivalent composites on a subsample of subjects [2].

Important achievements of this study were the findings that in rural cohorts the intraindividual standard deviation for energy nutrients is of the same order, or slightly higher, than the interindividual variation. This greatly complicates the analysis of relationships between dietary variables and other characteristics of the individuals concerned. More favorable conditions for analysis can be found by comparison of averages in contrasting populations using highly standardized methods.

Also, in rapidly changing societies, relevant changes in food intake were observed over time. In fact, in the two rural areas of Italy, the subjects of Montegiorgio now approach the dietary habits of the subjects of Crevalcore, though very different at the start in 1960. They were abandoning, in 31 years, the traditional Mediterranean diet [2].

In some rural cohorts, three days of dietary record survey can be enough at the group level. Seasonal variations in diet were in general small.

In addition to high cost and time requirements, the weighed record method has other limitations. The most relevant is the change of habitual diet due to being observed. We tried to reduce this disadvantage by asking the children in the family about the usual family diet.

Dietary History Method

Only in Zutphen (Netherlands), in 1960 and following years, was the dietary history method used on all subjects. Retrospectively, this was an excellent decision, because the relationship between individual diet and subsequent mortality from all, and specific causes of death, was thereby possible to study. In fact, at the fifth-year follow-up in 1965 in the two rural Italian cohorts, the dietary history method was used on 1536 men 45 to 64 years old [3]. Very interesting results were obtained on the relation between food and nutrient intakes and death from coronary heart disease, stroke, cancer, liver cirrhosis, and all causes [4].

But there are also limitations in the dietary history method. A very highly qualified interviewer is required; it has a high subjective component; the method concentrates on the regular dietary pattern, thereby missing irregularities; information on day-to-day variation in food and nutrient intake cannot be obtained; methodological errors in recording, coding, and processing of data are possible; and the data processing is time-consuming.

Recently, colleagues from Finland and the Netherlands made a useful improvement for the fat intake assessment.

To reduce or eliminate methodological errors, we set up a questionnaire for the dietary history method. In 85 forms, a very wide list of coded foods consumed at different meals is included. Four squares (A, B, C, D) are provided to indicate the quantity consumed. Four further squares follow to indicate daily, weekly, monthly, and yearly frequency of consumption. For the frequency of consumption of a given quantity during the specified time period, one to six squares are provided. Seasonings used are specified separately. To identify the usual portion, a photograph album or food model is used. Account is taken of foods eaten only seasonally.

The questionnaire is filled in by a dietitian, who asks the subject first to describe the composition of his usual daily meals. After checking, the forms are loaded onto the automatic document feeder of a color image scanner. The scanner is connected to the computer and the appropriate software provides the daily food and nutrient consumption individually or in homogeneous groups.

Validation of the dietary history method has been carried out by comparison with results from the weighed record method in three different seasons. The surveys were carried out on 16 subjects of Crevalcore and Montegiorgio at the 31st-year follow-up of the Seven Countries Study in 1991. The differences between the two methods were not statistically significant [2].

With this questionnaire, methodological errors are considerably reduced and the results can be obtained in a shorter time.

For the subsample of Rome railroad men, the food diary method for seven days was used in June–July 1969. We had gained enough experience with this method with Naples City Hall employees and it was more practical for this particular group of subjects. For a correct use of this method it is necessary to have knowledge of the composition of usual dishes consumed in the area of study.

Food Composition Tables—Vitamin Nutriture

During follow-ups and in the interval years we did intensive work on the validity of food composition tables used in Italy and on the vitamin nutritional status of some subjects. For protein, fatty acids, starch, and some unavailable carbohydrates, the mean of differences between values obtained by chemical analysis and values obtained by calculation with food composition tables was statistically significant [5].

Also for vitamin C, the food composition table we used did not prove adequate [6]. No food composition table can estimate the vitamin C content of cooked foods as eaten. A common correction factor for losses of vitamin C in cooking cannot be recommended. Similar difficulties with the use of food composition table data exist for vitamin A, calcium, and iron [7].

In 1970 and 1991, we also assessed the vitamin status of the subjects of dietary surveys. For thiamine, with use of the erythrocyte transketolase activity method, a rather low prevalence of malnutrition was observed both in 1970 and 1991. For riboflavin, with use of the erythrocyte glutathione reductase activity method, a higher prevalence of malnutrition was observed. In 1991, for example, the prevalence of β-carotene malnutrition was very high.

In general, the correlation between nutrient intake and nutritional status assessed biochemically was not high. The only valid way to assess vitamin and mineral nutriture is by biochemical methods. The methodology in the last few years is greatly improved [8].

Multiple Measurement Method

In order to evaluate the number of days of recorded intake required to obtain an estimate of the components of variance (the interindividual and the intraindividual variability), focusing on foods rather than nutrients, we recently developed an interesting method [9]. In a group of elderly persons surveyed for 3 nonconsecutive weeks, for each food examined, three statistical parameters were estimated: the variation between individuals, the intraindividual variation, and the mean of intakes. For each food item, the components of variance were estimated 20 times on food intake measures on the basis of the average of the first 2 days (the first time), and then adding the following days of collection, 1 day at a time until the 21st day of collection. The estimation of the mean and the inter- and intraindividual variation for milk at breakfast became stable after a few days of recorded intake. The same findings were found for other foods such as cereals. At lunch, the estimation of the mean and the inter- and intraindividual variation became stable after a few days of recorded intakes for cereals, vegetables, cheeses, fruits, potatoes, eggs, and meat. A rather similar situation was observed at dinner. By this method, a few days of food intake can be considered sufficient to obtain an estimate of the components of variance and of the mean for most of the food items.

Food Frequency Method

The food frequency method has become very common in recent years to address issues of usual diet in chronic diseases. Many questionnaires are available; the most recent is that of Willett, providing for optical reading. The main limitations of this questionnaire are: the limited number of food items, only one standard serving size is incorporated, and only nine compulsory frequency classes are available.

To avoid these limitations we have set up a semiquantitative, self-administered food frequency questionnaire. Based on the most common food habits, the questionnaire comprises on the left-hand side, in 16 printed forms, 93 food items grouped according to their nutritional characteristics. Three squares (A, B, C) indicating the quantity consumed are provided. Three further squares indicate daily, weekly, and monthly frequency consumption. For the frequency of consumption of a given quantity during the specified time interval, one to six squares are provided.

On the right-hand side, colored photographs of three (A, B, C) portions of 62 foods or dishes are displayed, to identify the usual portion consumed by the subject. The instructions for self-administration of the questionnaire are given at the beginning, with a form for sociodemographic data. Two extra printed forms for fat consumption and composition of daily meals are included at the end. For seasonal foods, a 33%–66% reduction of the three portions (A, B, C) is applied.

The subject has to fill in with a red pen the squares corresponding to the food portions and frequencies in the 16 printed forms. After checking, the 16 forms are loaded onto the automatic document feeder of a color image scanner. The scanner is connected to the computer and appropriate software provides the daily food and dish consumption individually or in 25 homogeneous groups.

The printed forms generally take 15 min to complete. The scanner reading and data processing are done in about 10 min.

This questionnaire was validated by comparison with nutrient intake obtained with the weighed record method for 7 days and with biochemical variables (24-h urine nitrogen, phosphorus, potassium, and sodium excretion; blood ascorbic acid and β-carotene levels). Statistically significant correlations were obtained for most nutrients, with the exception of blood ascorbic acid and β-carotene.

Camera Method

In order to assess the potential intake of food components and contaminants in a large group of individuals, we have used a "camera" method.

On about 15 000 students attending the university canteen in Perugia, we assessed food intake at lunch and dinner for 6 consecutive days in two different seasons (winter and spring) with a video camera.

The video cameras are located at the end of three distribution lines and record each tray marked with different alphabetic letters to identify the sex of the students. The leftovers were recorded at the end of the meal. The videocassettes were then watched on a TV video, and the foods and beverages chosen by students were registered on a special form and transferred to the computer for processing. For each student, 8 min for data recording, coding, and computing were required.

Videotel Method

In France, the SU.VI.MAX study has recently started. This is a national project coordinated by the Institut Scientifique et Technique de la Nutrition et de l'Alimentation, in Paris, to assess the effect of antioxidant vitamin and mineral supplementation on chronic disease incidence. The sample is 15000 subjects screened from about 100000 volunteers.

By means of videotel, each subject is asked every 2 months to transmit the food intake of the previous day. Each food has an identification code, and quantification is done by means of three photos appearing on the videotel screen, corresponding to three different portions of the food indicated with the letters B, D, and F. If the portion is smaller, intermediate, or larger, the subject can indicate this with letters A, C, E, and G.

The data collected are immediately elaborated and energy, carbohydrate, fat, and protein intake are transmitted online to the subject, along with the trend for the year. A preliminary validation study has already been performed. Further tests are in progress.

Conclusions

In conclusion, after many years of work with the Seven Countries Studies food intake assessment, we can say:

1. The use of the weighed record method on a subsample of subjects is still recommended to assess intra- and interindividual variability. In some cases the food diary method is preferred. No validation of this last method is at the moment available.
2. Concurrently, on all subjects, the dietary history method is also recommended. The two methods provide comparable results and their validity has been tested.
3. The food frequency method has some use, but valid results are limited to food intake only. In fact, the assessment of food items and dishes is limited and semiquantitative. The test of validity is satisfactory.
4. Validation of food composition tables with chemical analysis of food composites is compulsory. If this test is not satisfactory, we can rely only on chemical analysis of food composites.
5. Very promising are the camera method and the Videotel system for large-scale surveys.
6. Other methods based on recall cannot be recommended for all populations. In some of them unreliable results were obtained.
7. Nutritional status assessment is highly recommended, particularly for vitamins, minerals, and trace elements. The methodology has been greatly improved in the last few years. The use of nutrient intake to assess status is not sufficient.
8. In rapidly changing societies, the longitudinal assessment of food intake is highly recommended.

Acknowledgment. This work was supported by the Italian National Research Council (CNR) targeted project "Prevention and Control of Disease Factors," subproject "Nutrition," CNR contract nos. 92.00093 and 93.00657. PF41.

References

1. den Hartog C, Buzina R, Fidanza F, Keys A, Roine P (1968) Dietary studies and epidemiology of heart diseases. The Stichting tot wetenschapellijke op Voedings-gebied, The Hague, Netherlands
2. Alberti-Fidanza A, Alunni Paolacci C, Chiuchiu MP, Coli R, Fruttini D, Verducci G, Fidanza F (1994) Dietary studies on two rural Italian population groups of the Seven Countries Study. 1. Food and nutrient intake at the thirty-first year follow-up in 1991. Eur J Clin Nutr 48:85–91
3. Alberti-Fidanza A, Seccareccia F, Torsello F, Fidanza F (1988) Diet of two rural population groups of middle-aged men in Italy. Int J Vit Nutr Res 58:442–451
4. Farchi G, Mariotti S, Menotti A , Seccareccia F, Torsello S, Fidanza F (1989) Diet and 20-year mortality in two rural population groups of middle-aged men in Italy. Am J Clin Nutr 50:1095–1103
5. Alberti-Fidanza A, Alunni Paolacci C, Chiuchiu MP, Coli R, Parretta MG, Verducci G, Fidanza F (1994) Dietary studies on two rural population groups of the Seven Countries Study. 2. Concurrent validation of protein, fat and carbohydrate intake. Eur J Clin Nutr 48:92–96
6. Fidanza F, Senin-Zanetti P (1971) Comparison of chemical analysis and calculated values of vitamin C consumed by population groups of two rural areas of Italy. Int J Vit Nutr Res 41:307–312
7. Fidanza F (1974) Sources of error in dietary surveys. Bibl Nutr Diet 20:105–113
8. Fidanza F (ed) (1991) Nutritional status assessment. Chapman and Hall, London
9. Borrelli R, Simonetti MS, Fidanza F (1992) Inter- and intraindividual variability in food intake of elderly people in Perugia (Italy). Br J Nutr 68:3–10

Discussion

D. Kromhout: Your data on legumes showed a very large intraindividual variation. It is also important to have a good reference category. For instance, in The Netherlands we have done an analysis in which we can compare legume users and nonusers, which allows us to show associations. Thus, intraindividual variation is of importance, but if you can find a group of nonusers you are in a very good situation. These are separate issues in my point of view.

F. Fidanza: Well, I am not very happy with epidemiological criteria considering extremes of users and nonusers. I am doing nutritional epidemiology, yes, but with a different approach.

Part 3
Recent Trends in Cardiovascular Diseases and Risk Factors in the Seven Countries Study

Recent Trends in Cardiovascular Disease and Risk Factors in the Seven Countries Study: Japan

YOSHINORI KOGA, RYUICHI HASHIMOTO, HISASHI ADACHI,
MAKOTO TSURUTA, HIROMI TASHIRO, and HIRONORI TOSHIMA

Summary. Rapid socioeconomic developments in Japan since the beginning of the Seven Countries Study in 1958 have brought remarkable changes in lifestyles and dietary patterns. Time trends in nutrient intake, risk factors, and cardiovascular disease (CVD) mortality and morbidity have been monitored in men aged 40–64 in a Japanese cohort of the Seven Countries Study, in Tanushimaru, a typical farming town on Kyushu Island.

The total daily calorie intake decreased from 2837 Kcal in 1958 to 2228 Kcal in 1968, and remained stable thereafter. The carbohydrate intake in percentage of total daily calories decreased markedly, from 78.1% in 1958 to 60.6% in 1989, in contrast to large increases during this period in protein intake (from 10.9% to 15.6%) and fat intake (from 5.3% to 21.6%).

The mean serum cholesterol level was 150 ± 41 mg/dl in 1958 (Keys method), and rapidly increased to 161 ± 32 in 1977 and to 188 ± 37 mg/dl in 1989 (enzymatic method). The frequency of overweight (body mass index exceeding 26) was 8% in 1958, and gradually increased to 11% in 1977 and to 18% in 1989. The frequency of diastolic hypertension (≥ 95 mmHg) gradually increased from 8% in 1958 to 20% in 1982, and then declined to 13% in 1989. The frequency of isolated systolic hypertension also decreased steadily to 1989. The percentage of smokers decreased from 69% in 1958 to 55% in 1989.

The 15-year mortality and incidence rates for stroke and myocardial infarction were compared between two separate cohorts in Tanushimaru, the first sampled in 1958 and the second in 1977. Age-adjusted death rate from all causes declined from 17.6 to 7.4/1000 per year. Stroke mortality declined dramatically from 4.6 to 0.8/1000 per year, while no appreciable change occurred in the death rate from myocardial infarction (0.3 to 0.5/1000 per year) or sudden deaths (0.4 to 0.6/1000 per year). Stroke incidence declined from 6.7 to 4.4/1000 per year, but no appreciable trend was observed in the incidence of myocardial infarction (0.9 to 1.2/1000 per year).

The large changes in dietary patterns and lifestyles in Tanushimaru since 1958 have been associated with a remarkable reduction in stroke, but no increase in myocardial infarction. It is suggested that dietary changes in Tanushimaru in the last 30 years have contributed to the prevention of cardiovascular diseases. Continuation of the rapid increase in dietary fat calories could, however, change this favorable picture.

Key words. Nutrient intake—Food consumption—Risk factors—Mortality and morbidity trends—Stroke—Myocardial infarction

Introduction

At the beginning of the Seven Countries Study in 1958, Japanese cohorts of Tanushimaru and Ushibuka presented with the lowest saturated fat intake and levels of serum cholesterol, and among the lowest incidence rates of coronary heart disease [1].

Subsequently, Japan has experienced dramatic changes in lifestyle and eating patterns associated with socioeconomic development [2]. Associated mortality trends have occurred with a rapid decrease in pulmonary tuberculosis, a rise and subsequent fall in stroke deaths, and a continuing decline in deaths from malignant neoplasms. Though the crude death rate from all heart diseases has been increasing, the age-adjusted rate has remained constant [3]. These changes in death rates are associated with considerable prolongation of estimates of life expectancy in Japanese, exceeding 76 years in men and 82 in women, in 1992 [3].

The aim of this report is to describe time trends in eating patterns, lifestyles, and risk factors in Tanushimaru and to discuss how these transitions have influenced coronary heart disease and stroke mortality and morbidity.

Subjects and Methods

Trends in nutritional patterns, risk factors, and cardiovascular disease mortality and morbidity have been monitored in a typical farming town, Tanushimaru, located on Kyushu, the southwestern island of Japan. The first survey was begun in 1958 as a Japanese cohort of the Seven Countries Study. All men (*n* = 639) aged 40–64 years who were born and had lived in the Chikuyo area of Tanushimaru were enrolled, with a response rate of 100%. The Japanese cohorts of the Seven Countries Study included men over age 60, in addition to the standard cohorts of men aged 40–59 years.

In 1968, 10 years after the first survey, 543 men of the first cohort aged 50–74 received a standardized follow-up examination. In 1977, an independent second cohort was identified, enrolling 573 men aged 40–64 years in the same district of Tanushimaru. This newly drawn cross-sectional survey (response rate 90.1%) included some who participated in the first survey in 1958. Third and fourth cross-sectional surveys were conducted in 1982 and 1989 in the same district of Tanushimaru for all men aged 40–64 years. There were 602 participants in 1982 and 752 in 1989, with a response rate of 77% and 89%, respectively. The third and fourth cohorts added women aged 40–64 living in the same district, 747 in 1982 (response rate 81%) and 707 in 1989 (response rate 70%).

Each cross-sectional survey was conducted using the common protocol described in detail by Keys and associates [1,4]. The measurements included (a) age; (b) occupation; (c) eating patterns as determined by 24-h dietary recall; (d) salt intake estimation by the amount of soup consumed; (e) area of arable land worked and physical work; (f) family history; (g) alcohol drinking and smoking; (h) body size; (i) physical examination; (j) blood pressure; (k) electrocardiogram and exercise stress test (Master's two-step method); (l) serum cholesterol by the Keys method in 1958 and 1968 and by the enzymatic method in 1977, 1982, and 1989; and (m) serum lipoproteins (Swahn's method). Although new measurements were added in the second to fourth surveys, including serum protein, optic fundi, HDL-cholesterol, etc., the same protocol was followed.

Systematic follow-up surveys of all-causes deaths and incidence and death rate for cardiovascular diseases were carried out for cohort 1 (entry 1958) and cohort 2 (entry 1977). Diagnoses and disease classification were made according to the protocol of the Seven Countries Study [1]. Fifteen-year mortality and morbidity are presented here.

Results and Discussion

Changes in Nutritional Patterns

The serial changes in nutrient intake in Tanushimaru are summarized in Fig. 1. In 1958, the total daily calorie intake was 2837 Kcal, and 78% was derived from carbohydrates. Total daily calorie intake decreased to 2228 Kcal in 1968, and remained stable thereafter. However, there was a progressive decrease in intake of carbohydrates, from 78% in 1958 to 61% in 1989, and a progressive increase in intake of fat calories, from 5% to 22%, and protein, from 11% to 16%.

These changes in food consumption, assessed by 24-h recall, are presented in Fig. 2. Rice consumption decreased dramatically, from 593 g/day in 1958 to 299 g/day in 1977 and 290 g/day in 1982, and fell to 232 g/day in 1989. There have been progressive increases in consumption of meats, fish and shellfish, and milk.

The reduction of total calorie intake can be attributed in part to the dramatic changes in working conditions of farming in Japan, from traditional heavy physical labor to the current use of automated farming machines. Reduced walking due to the wider use of automobiles is an additional factor. Departure from the traditional Japanese diet, high in salt and carbohydrate while low in fat and protein, toward Western foods and eating patterns, has further contributed to these major trends.

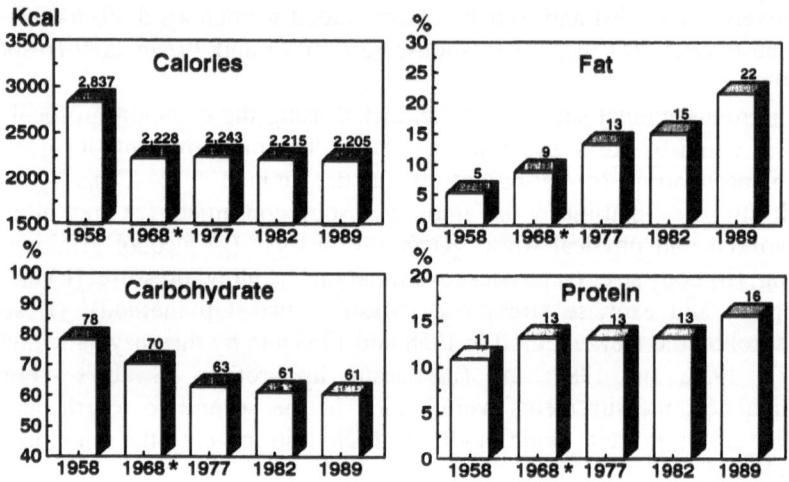

Fig. 1. Time trends in total daily calories and percent calories from fat, carbohydrate, and protein in Tanushimaru men aged 40–64 years (50–64 years in 1968[*]). Numbers are average values from 24-h recall

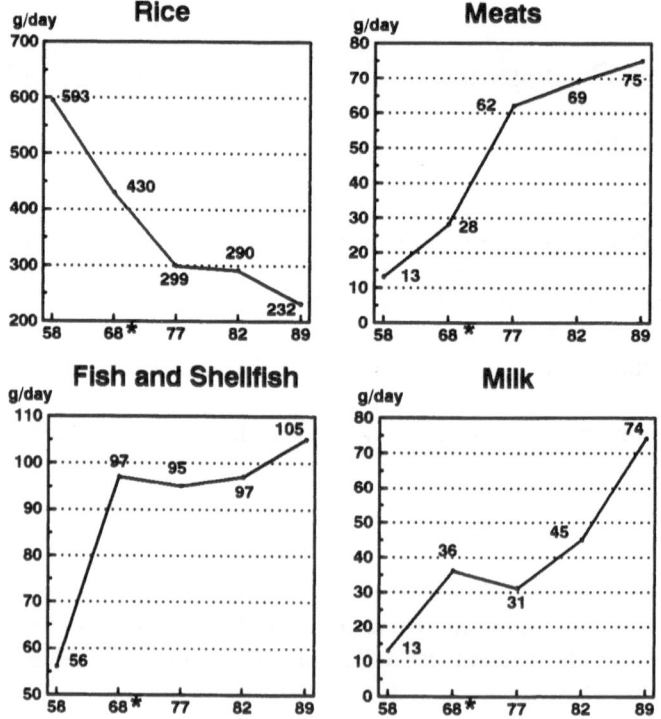

Fig. 2. Time trends in food consumption (g/day) in Tanushimaru men aged 40–64 years (50–64 years in 1968[*]). Numbers are average values, from 24-h recall

Changes in Risk Factors

The reduction of daily physical activity likely influenced as well the progressive increase in the sum of skinfold thickness in all age groups (Fig. 3). The frequency of overweight defined by body mass index exceeding 26 was 7.4% in 1958, and gradually increased to 9.5% in 1977, and 18.1% in 1989.

These changes in eating patterns and lifestyles have probably contributed to the progressive increases in average serum cholesterol levels (Fig. 4), from 150 ± 41 mg/dl in 1958 (Keys method) to 161 ± 32 in 1977 and 188 ± 37 in 1989 (enzymatic method). The serum cholesterol levels in women aged 40 to 64 were higher than those in men, 192 ± 35 mg/dl in 1982 and 206 ± 40 in 1989.

The prevalence of diastolic hypertension (≥95 mmHg) increased from 8% in 1958 to a peak of 20% in 1982 (Fig. 5). This trend coincided with a parallel increase in obesity. The subsequent decline in diastolic hypertension in 1989 may be attributed in part to the wide application of antihypertensive medications. The frequency of isolated systolic hypertension decreased up until 1989.

Figure 6 shows the percentage of smokers. Despite a slight decline, smoking among men is still high in Japan.

Trends of Cardiovascular Mortality and Morbidity in Tanushimaru

Table 1 describes the 15-year mortality rates and incidence of stroke and myocardial infarction, comparing two cohorts of Tanushimaru; cohort 1, the original cohort of the Seven Countries, from 1958 until 1973, and cohort 2, a

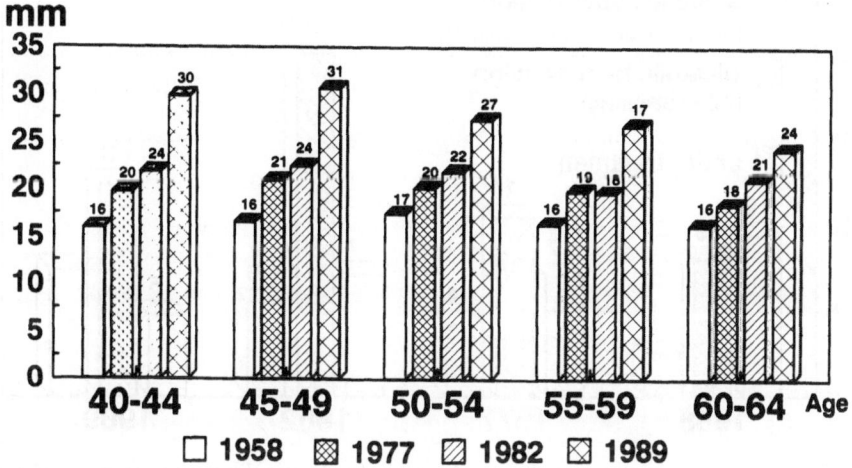

Fig. 3. Time trends in skinfold thickness (over the triceps muscle plus over the tip of the scapula) in Tanushimaru men of the five age groups. Numbers are average values

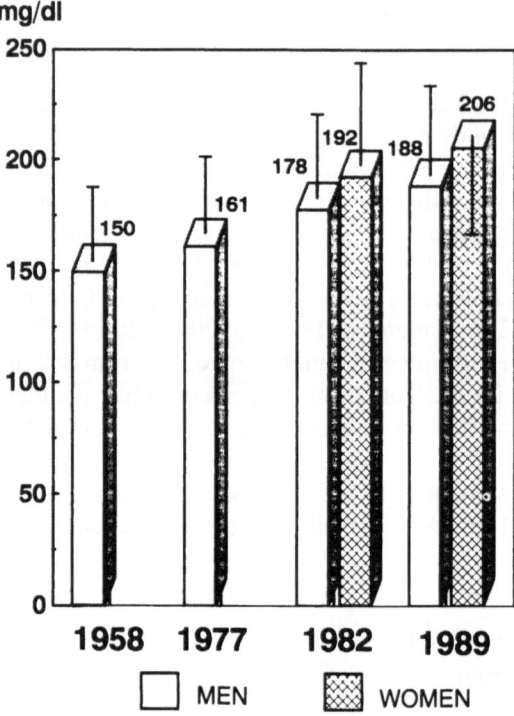

Fig. 4. Time trends in serum cholesterol levels in Tanushimaru men aged 40–64 years. The values for women of the same ages in 1982 and 1989 are also presented. Numbers are average values; bars indicate standard deviations

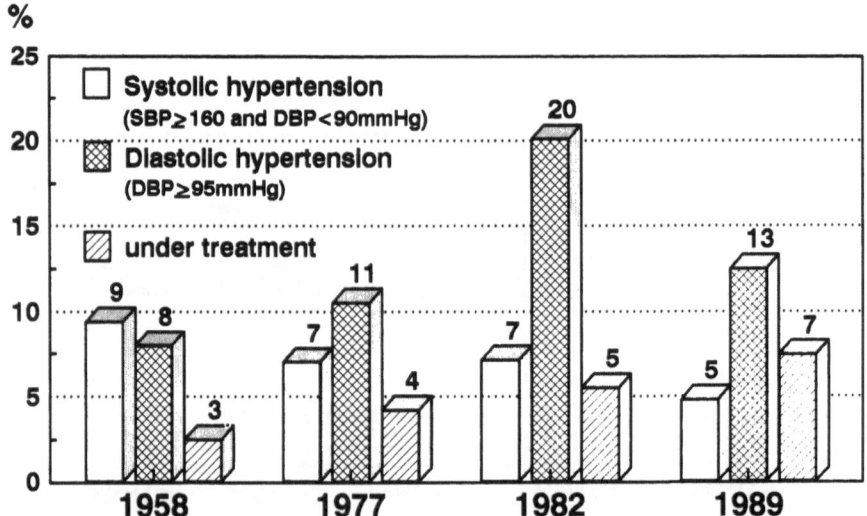

Fig. 5. Time trends in the prevalence of systolic and diastolic hypertension, and percentages of those receiving antihypertensive medication, in Tanushimaru men aged 40–64 years

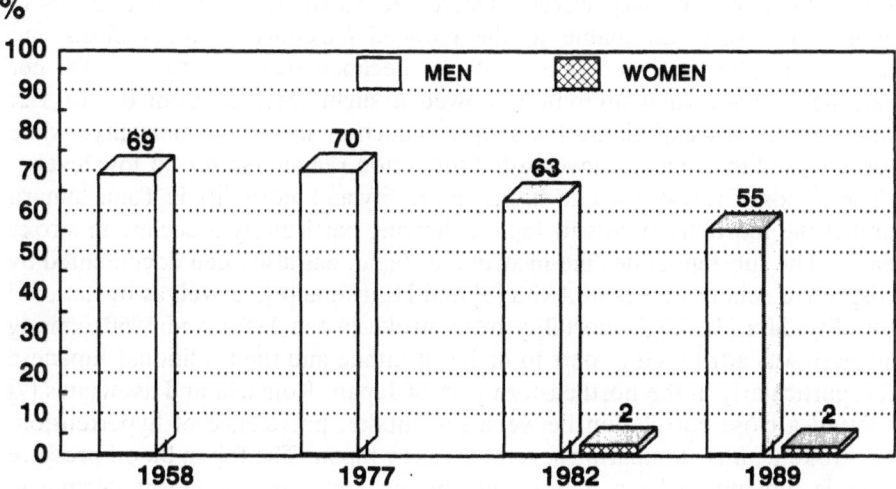

Fig. 6. Time trends in percentage of smokers in Tanushimaru men aged 40–64 years. The percentage for women of the same ages in 1982 and 1989 are also presented

Table 1. Fifteen-year mortality and incidence of stroke and myocardial infarction in two cohorts of Tanushimaru men aged 40–64 at entry[a].

	Cohort 1 1958–1973 ($n = 636$)	Cohort 2 1977–1992 ($n = 567$)
Mortality		
Stroke	44 (4.6)	7 (0.8)
Myocardial infarction	3 (0.3)	4 (0.5)
Sudden death	4 (0.4)	5 (0.6)
Cancer	45 (4.7)	29 (3.4)
Others	72 (7.6)	18 (2.1)
Total	168 (17.6)	63 (7.4)
Incidence		
Stroke	64 (6.7)	37 (4.4)
Hemorrhage	22 (2.3)	17 (2.0)
Infarction	38 (4.0)	14 (1.7)
Unclassified	4 (0.4)	6 (0.7)
Myocardial infarction	9 (0.9)	10 (1.2)

[a] Number of deaths or incidence rates per 1000 persons per year.

new cross-sectional survey started in 1977 and followed until 1992. The stroke mortality in cohort 1 was 4.6/1000 per year, but this fell drastically to 0.8/1000 per year in cohort 2. Mortality rates for myocardial infarction, sudden death, and cancer were relatively stable, changing from 0.3 to 0.5, 0.4 to 0.6, and 4.7

to 3.4/1000 per year, respectively. Decreased mortality from other causes in cohort 2 is largely ascribable to the reduced incidence of tuberculosis and pneumonia. The incidence rate of stroke declined from 6.7 to 4.4/1000 per year, while myocardial infarction showed a slight increase from 0.9 to 1.2. Tanushimaru has experienced a major reduction in stroke mortality, while mortality and incidence of myocardial infarction remain, so far, at low levels.

The trends of cardiovascular disease mortality and morbidity in Tanushimaru parallel the mortality trends in Japan, showing particularly a decline in stroke deaths. The substantial decline in stroke in Japan has also been documented by prospective cohort studies in Akita [5] and Hisayama [6], as well as by national mortality data [3]. High mortality from stroke in the 1950s and 1960s among Japanese was attributed in part to high salt intake and the traditional Japanese diet, particularly in the northeastern part of Japan. Komachi and associates [7] reported a close correlation between salt intake, prevalence of hypertension, and stroke deaths, comparing several areas in Japan. The fall in blood pressure levels is thought to be a major contributing factor in the recent decline in stroke in Japan [8].

Alternatively, low fat intake and low serum cholesterol level, averaging 150 to 170 mg/dl in the 1950s and 1960s, were considered an additional risk factor for cerebral hemorrhage in the Akita study of Inada and associates [9]. In Tanushimaru and Ushibuka, Kimura and associates [10] reported an inverse association of serum albumin and cerebral hemorrhage. An increase in protein and/or animal fat consumption could explain the decline in stroke in Japan, although the hypothesis is controversial and requires further study [11].

Mortality and morbidity trends for myocardial infarction in Tanushimaru are consistent with the Hisayama Study [6], another population survey from Kyushu Island which included systematic autopsy examinations to differentiate cerebral hemorrhage from infarction. In that study, there was no evidence of an increase in myocardial infarction incidence between two 10-year study periods; cohort 1, from 1961 to 1970, and cohort 2, from 1974 to 1983. In a northern Japan study in Akita [5], where the incidence of stroke was known to be high, a remarkable decline in stroke incidence was found, but no increase in that of myocardial infarction. The Akita study was conducted in a farming community, and the changing pattern of nutrient intake was similar to the experience in Tanushimaru, with considerable increases in fat and protein intake and decreases in carbohydrate and salt intakes.

It should be noted, however, that these studies, including the Tanushimaru study, were conducted in rural Japan. With economic development, Japanese urban populations are now involved much more in westernized lifestyles and eating patterns. It is thus quite possible that the urban consumption, particularly of animal products, is considerably higher than the rural, leading to much higher average cholesterol levels. However, few epidemiological studies have been conducted in large cities because of the difficulty of long-term follow-up in such mobile populations.

Konishi and associates [12] have monitored the incidence of cardiovascular disease in desk workers of several large companies in Osaka since 1965. Along with a considerable decrease in stroke incidence they also noted a trend of increasing coronary heart disease incidence, although the differences were not statistically significant. In that cohort, the latest mean serum cholesterol level was around 180–200 mg/dl. The upward trend for coronary heart disease in Osaka was not explained by higher cholesterol levels alone, and other risk factors were considered, such as overwork, stress, smoking, and decreased physical exercise.

The mortality trends for "heart disease" in Japan [3] are shown in Fig. 7. The crude death rate from coronary heart disease increased until 1970, but remained stable thereafter. The age-corrected death rate from coronary heart disease is even decreasing. This finding, however, must be interpreted with caution. Attention should be paid to the rapid increase in the death rate from "other heart diseases" and the possibility that death from heart attack has been reported in generic terms as "acute heart failure" on the death certificate and thus is classified as "other heart disease" instead of coronary heart disease. In the Tokyo metropolitan area, the Tokyo Medical Examiner's Office has conducted systematic autopsy examinations on victims of sudden death to identify the exact cause of death [13]. Among 839 cases of sudden death autopsied between January and December 1989, 418 cases (49.8%) were found to be due to coronary heart disease. This implies strongly that the coronary death rate is underestimated in Japan and might be corrected upwards, between the two lines of Fig. 7.

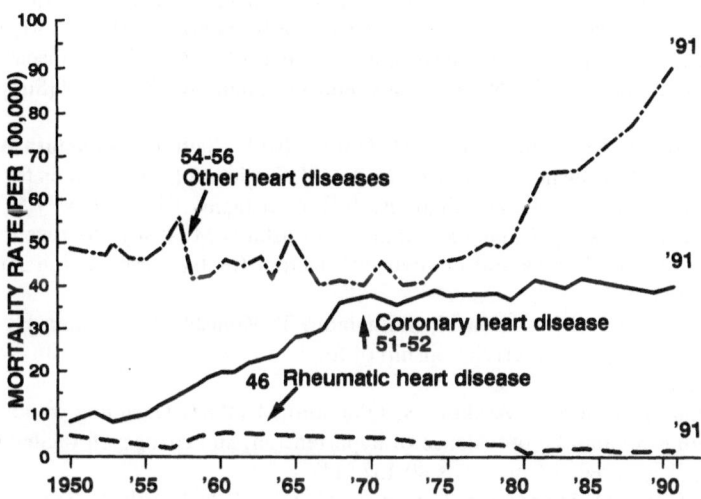

Fig. 7. Trends in cardiac disease mortality (crude death rates) in Japan. Data from [3]

In our clinical experience in Kurume, the number of patients with myocardial infarction has increased substantially both in the coronary care unit and in the cardiology ward. Recent advances in management of coronary patients may have improved survival and kept many long-term patients alive, thus preventing an increase in the death rate. This may be responsible for the inconsistent findings between clinical experience and the statistics from death certificates. However, it is also true that the Japanese are now enjoying the greatest longevity in the world.

We conclude that the changed composition of the Japanese diet has probably improved health and reduced stroke rates. However, careful surveillance is needed in the future because of the increasing intake of fats, especially saturated fatty acids, with the potential of a modern epidemic of coronary disease in Japan.

References

1. Keys A, Aravanis C, Blackburn H, Buzina R, Djordjević BS, Dontas AS, Fidanza F, Karvonen MJ, Kimura N, Menotti A, Mohacek A, Nedeljković S, Puddu V, Punsar S, Taylor HL, van Buchem FSP (1980) Seven Countries Study. A multivariate analysis of death and coronary heart disease. Harvard University Press, Cambridge, Mass.
2. Toshima H, Tashiro H, Sumie M, Koga Y, Kimura N (1984) Nutritional prevention of cardiovascular disease. In: Lovenberg W, Yamori Y (eds) Changes in risk factors and cardiovascular mortality and morbidity within Tanushimaru 1958–1982. Academic Press, New York, pp 203–210
3. Ministry of Health and Welfare of Japan (1993) Health Welfare Stat 40:43–87
4. Keys A, Aravanis C, Blackburn H, van Buchem FSP, Buzina R, Djordjević BS, Dontas AS, Fidanza F, Karvonen MJ, Kimura N, Lekos D, Menotti M, Puddu V, Taylor HL (1966) Epidemiological studies related to coronary heart disease: characteristics of men aged 40–59 in Seven Countries. Acta Med Scand 460[Suppl 180]:1–392
5. Shimamoto T, Komachi Y, Inada H, Doi M, Iso H, Saitou S, Kitamura A, Iida M, Konishi M, Nakanishi N, Terao A, Naitou Y, Kojima S (1989) Trends for coronary heart disease and stroke and their risk factors in Japan. Circulation 79:503–515
6. Ueda K, Arakawa J, Tanaka K, Omae T, Fujishima M (1990) The recent trends of atherosclerotic diseases and of their risk factors (in Japanese). J Jpn Atheroscler Soc 18:125–131
7. Komachi Y, Iida M, Ozawa H, Shimamoto T, Konishi M, Ueshima H, Goda N, Furukawa M (1975) Interrelationship of food and stroke in Japan. Ann Rep Center Adult Dis Osaka 15:82–93
8. Ueshima H, Tatara K, Asakura S, Okamoto M (1987) Declining trends in blood pressure level and the prevalence of hypertension, and changes in related factors in Japan, 1956–1980. J Chron Dis 40:137–147
9. Inada H, Iida M, Shimamoto T, Konishi M, Doi M, Nakanishi N, Terao A, Naitou Y, Iso H, Fukuuti K, Saitou S, Kitamura A, Kojima S, Funaki M, Komachi Y (1986) Morbidity trends in stroke and ischemic heart disease and changes in the

major risk factors for stroke in rural farming area in Akita prefecture, Japan (in Japanese with English abstract). Jpn J Pub Health 22:387–397

10. Kimura N, Toshima H, Nakayama Y, Takayama K, Tashiro H, Takagi M (1979) Fifteen-year follow-up population survey on stroke: A multivariate analysis of the risk of stroke in farmers of Tanushimaru and fishermen of Ushibuka. In: Yamori Y, Lovenberg W, Freid ED (eds) Prophylactic approach to hypertensive diseases. Raven, New York, pp 505–510

11. Blackburn H, Jacobs DR (1989) The ongoing natural experiment of cardiovascular diseases in Japan. Circulation 79:718–720

12. Konishi M, Iida M, Naitou M, Terao A, Kiyama M, Kojima S, Shimamoto T, Doi M, Komachi Y (1987) Studies on the relationship between the trends of serum total cholesterol level and the incidence of cerebro-cardiovascular diseases based on the follow-up studies in Akita and Osaka—with a special reference to the optimal serum total cholesterol level preventing cerebral hemorrhage and coronary heart disease (in Japanese with English abstract). J Jpn Atheroscler Soc 15:1115–1123

13. Tokudomi S, Yanaguchi Y (1989) Analysis of the causes of unexpected acute death of autopsied cases. J Clin Sci 25:671–678

Discussion

A. Keys: When, in 1956, Margaret and I were here in Japan with Dr. Paul Dudley White, our Japanese hosts could not find a single case of coronary heart disease. The chief pathologist at the medical school showed us a fascinating case, to him, of acute myocardial infarction in a Japanese doctor who had practiced 20 years in the United States. The pathologist said he had never seen anything like it before, the coronary arteries showing marked atherosclerosis. I think things may have changed now.

R. Beaglehole: I wonder if you could clarify the situation with regard to other heart disease. I have seen data suggesting that other heart disease death rates are going down in Japan. Are these age-standardized rates?

Y. Koga: These are crude rates. Age-corrected rates of other heart disease are also decreasing.

H. Ueshima: Age-adjusted, all heart disease mortality has generallly been declining in Japan since 1970. The category "other heart disease" is also declining in Japan.

Y. Koga: There must be other reasons for the decline in CHD which we must look for, as in case-fatality. I think the skill in management of heart disease is improving and case fatality is decreasing rapidly in Japan. So I think that incidence is going up but, admittedly, we have yet to establish that definitely.

D. Jacobs: Dr. Koga, I want to pursue the question of the "true" cause of heart failure in Japan. Recently, Dr. Baba analyzed police records and other available data and concluded that there were not many hidden cases of coronary heart disease in the heart failure category of death certificates in Japan. I wonder if you know about that study and have an opinion about it?

Y. Koga: I do not know those data, but it may depend on the region. For example, a recent study in the Kyoto area indicated that 70% of sudden deaths were of coronary origin. So it depends a great deal on the region we are dealing with and what population—rural versus urban, for example.

C. Kawai: I can add data from the Tokyo coroner's office which includes more than 600 sudden deaths. These data revealed that 50% of 600 sudden death cases were afflicted with ischemic heart disease.

Recent Trends in Cardiovascular Disease and Risk Factors: Yugoslavia

Srecko I. Nedeljković, miodrag Č. Ostojić,
Milija R. Vukotić, and Miodrag Z. Grujić

Summary. This paper presents trends from demographic and health statistics data of the former Yugoslavia (fYU) and recently of the Federal Republic of Yugoslavia (RYU). The war and economic depression in the last 3 years have dramatically increased rates of diseases, injuries and deaths. Until recently, from 1950 to 1991, there had been a steady increase of life expectancy for fYU. According to the 1992 *World Health Statistics Annual*, fYU, compared to the Seven Countries and Hungary, has now reached high rates of cardiovascular disease (CVD) deaths on the same order as in the USA, Italy, Greece, and the Netherlands, but lower than in Finland and in Hungary. However, in Vojvodina, the northern province of Serbia, CVD deaths were as frequent as in Hungary. Trends in CVD deaths increased in fYU between the 1960s and 1980, and then stabilized with a slight decline until 1990. However, according to the 1991–1992 data for Central Serbia and Vojvodina, rates for all-cause and CVD deaths are dramatically increasing. In fYU, RYU, and particularly in Central Serbia and Vojvodina, the proportional contributions of CVD deaths to all-cause deaths is greater than 50% in men and 60% in women. In the Serbian part of the Seven Countries Study, after 25 years of follow-up of men aged 40–59 at entry, the best survival was found for Belgrade University professors, although they died proportionally more from CVD. The highest age-adjusted 25-year mortality (among the highest in the Seven Countries Study) was observed in Zrenjanin, a town representative of Vojvodina. The Zrenjanin cohort was characterized by major increases of risk factors over the first 10 years, especially of serum cholesterol and blood pressure; these were real changes and not only due to aging.

Key words. Yugoslavia—Vojvodina—CVD mortality—All-cause deaths— Risk factors—Life expectancy

Introduction

Until early 1992, the former Yugoslavia (fYU) functioned as a federal state before breaking into new states still in evolution: Slovenia, Croatia, Bosnia, and Herzegovina, the former republic of Macedonia, and the Federal Republic of Yugoslavia (RYU), which includes the republics of Montenegro and Serbia and the provinces of Vojvodina and Kosovo-Metohija (Kosmet).

Until 1991, when the last fYU census was held, demographic and health statistics were uniformly carried out and centralized, providing data for the whole fYU [1,2]. Demographic changes in fYU, over the last 50 years have been toward an increase in the population, although with a relatively greater decrease of birth rates versus mortality, bringing down the population growth rate nearly to zero. In the last 3 years in fYU, there has been an intense migration approaching 2 million displaced persons, and there are no exact data on loss of lives due to war injuries, malnutrition, and disease. This presents serious limitations to the study of recent trends in CVD deaths and risk factors. Psychosocial and economic factors are also emerging as an independent hazard for general and cardiovascular health in most fYU territories.

On the basis of data from the 1992 *World Health Statistics Annual* [3], rates of CVD and all-cause mortality in fYU for the year 1990 are compared to data from Hungary and the other countries in which the Seven Countries Study (SCS) was conducted. For analysis of trends of CVD and all-cause deaths in the interval between 1980–1992, data have been provided by the Federal Institute of Statistics [1] and from a monograph on Serbian mortality [4].

SCS data have also been used here for study of risk factor and CVD mortality trends in the Serbian part of the SCS [5–9].

Demographic Trends in Former Yugoslavia

Censuses were carried out in the former Yugoslavia in 1921, 1931, 1948, 1953, 1961, 1971, 1981, and 1991. Population growth rates constantly decreased, although the absolute number of fYU inhabitants rose from 15 842 000 in 1948 to 23 476 000 in 1991.

After the breakup of fYU in early 1992, the Federal Republic of Yugoslavia (RYU), according to the census of 1991, had a total population of 10 409 000, of which 9 792 000 were in Serbia and 617 000 in Montenegro.

Looking at data in Figure 1 for the interval 1921–1990, the fYU population was undergoing a relative decrease in live births greater than the relative decline in mortality, reaching a natural growth rate of 5.2 per 1000.

Especially serious consequences have been observed in the northern Serbian province of Vojvodina, in which the live birth rate of 11.2/1000 fell below the mortality rate of 12.3/1000, a trend observed there since 1986. On the other side, in the Serbian province of Kosmet, birth rates have been, through many decades, around 30/1000, among the worlds highest.

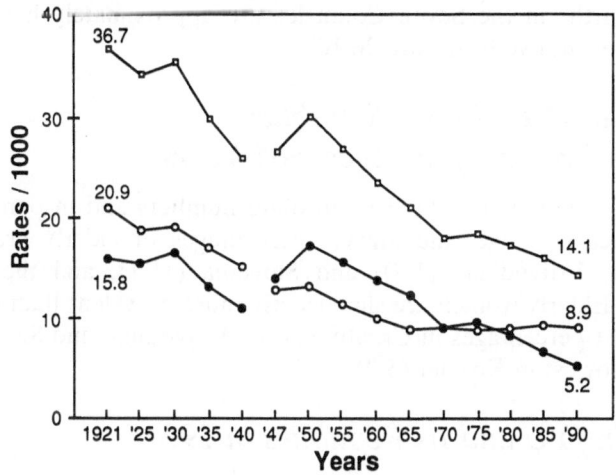

Fig. 1. Natality, mortality, and growth rate trends 1921–1990 in former Yugoslavia. *Squares*, live births; *open circles*, deaths; *closed circles*, growth rate

Demographic Changes in fYU and in the Seven Countries

According to the 1992 *World Health Statistics Annual* [3], in countries with market economies and in developing countries, demographic changes from 1990 to 1995 show an increase of elderly people ≥65 years, a decrease of the growth rate under 1/100, a decrease of live births under 14/1000, and relatively low death rates, around 9/1000. Moreover, mortality rates under age 5 were low, saving more babies and children due to new knowledge in perinatal and infant care.

In comparison with the other Seven Countries (Table 1) in 1990, fYU had a low percentage of elderly ≥65 years (9.8%), while Italy was on top with

Table 1. Population growth rate, natality, and mortality, 1992 estimate for 1990 to 1995, Seven Countries.

Country	Population (in thousands)	≥65 years Age (%)	Growth rate (per 100)	Live births nat. (per 1000)	Deaths (per 1000)
United States	255 159	12.6	1.0	15.9	8.9
Finland	5 008	13.6	0.3	12.8	10.2
Greece	10 182	14.4	0.3	10.4	9.8
Italy	57 782	14.7	0.1	10.0	10.1
Netherlands	15 158	12.8	0.7	13.7	8.7
Japan	124 491	12.5	0.4	11.2	7.5
f. Yugoslavia	23 949	9.8	0.3	14.1	9.5
Whole world	5 479 046	6.3	1.7	26.0	9.2

Data from [3].

14.7%. Live births in the Seven Countries are approximately half that elsewhere, where mean live births are 26/1000.

Population of fYU, Its Six Republics, and Serbian Provinces, at Ages >65 Years

Observing the population of fYU in absolute numbers and in percentages of elderly ≥65 years of age, the highest percentages of elderly are found in Croatia (11.8), Vojvodina (11.7), and Slovenia (11.1), and the lowest in Kosmet (4.6). Elderly women are significantly more prevalent than men, again with the highest percentages in Croatia (14.5), Vojvodina, and Slovenia (both 13.9) and the lowest in Kosmet (5.2).

Longevity in fYU and Its Republics in 1990

Longevity at birth increased in the two decades before 1990 in fYU and in all republics, with an average of 65.4 years for all of fYU in 1970 up to 69.1 in 1990 for men, and from 70.2 to 74.9 for women (Fig. 2). Women live on average 5 years longer. The greatest life expectancy up to 1990 was in the republics of Montenegro and Slovenia. Life expectancy estimates for the new RYU (Montenegro and Serbia) indicate that women have had much greater longevity than men in the long period from 1950 to 1991.

Life Expectancy and Chances of Dying from CVD

For this comparison, an extract of data from the 1992 *World Health Statistics Annual* [3] was used to show life expectancy and chances of dying from CVD in men at ages of 45 and 65 years, in all of the Seven Countries (Table 2). For

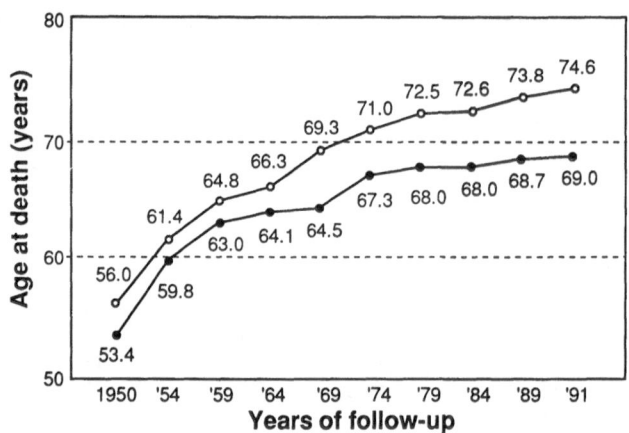

Fig. 2. Expected age at death of women (*open circles*) and men (*closed circles*), 1950–1991. Republic of Yugoslavia (Montenegro and Serbia)

Table 2. Life expectancy of men at ages 45 and 65 and chances of dying from malignancies, CVD, CHF, and cerebrovascular diseases in the Seven Countries.

Country	Age (years)	Life expectancy (years)	Chances of death (per 1000) from:			
			Malignancies	CVD	CHF + CM	Cerebrovascular
United States	45	30.8	248.2	469.9	368.8	62.3
1989	65	15.3	232.0	489.0	379.2	69.1
Finland	45	29.6	214.3	517.4	373.3	109.2
1991	65	14.1	212.0	533.4	374.2	121.4
Netherlands	45	31.0	301.2	411.7	288.9	81.8
1990	65	14.4	285.2	418.7	285.9	89.1
Italy	45	31.2	288.4	433.3	247.2	128.5
1989	65	15.0	258.2	461.8	254.4	143.0
Greece	45	32.4	234.0	514.1	320.8	171.5
1990	65	15.8	211.2	532.1	320.5	188.7
Japan	45	33.3	267.5	364.1	204.9	138.3
1991	65	16.6	244.7	380.0	213.6	144.0
f.Yugoslavia	45	28.4	186.7	546.1	344.4	144.1
1990	65	13.6	153.2	599.4	369.7	159.4

CVD, cardiovascular disease; CHF, congestive heart failure; CM, cardiomyopathy.
Data from [3].

fYU, life expectancy in 1990 was the lowest and the risk of eventually dying from CVD the highest of all the Seven Countries for both 45-year-old men (546.1 per 1000) and 65-year-old men (599.4 per 1000). As expected, the chance of eventually dying from CVD was also very high for men in Finland, but also, unexpectedly, for men in Greece. The risk of cerebrovascular disease death is high in Greece, and also in Yugoslavia. Of all the Seven Countries, Japanese men have the best life expectancy; men age 45 are expected to live until 78.3 years, and men age 65 until 81.6 years. Japanese men at ages 45 and 65 years also have the lowest chance, among all Seven Countries men, to die from CVD, at rates of 364.1 and 380.0 per 1000, respectively, though their risk of cerebrovascular disease death remains high.

All-cause and Specific Cardiovascular Mortality in fYU (1990) and the Seven Countries Plus Hungary

This presentation includes Hungary because of the many cultural and socioeconomic ties and similarities with Vojvodina (Zrenjanin) and Slavonia, two cohorts of the SCS. In 1991 WHO [3] reported the highest cardiovascular mortality in Hungary, followed by Greece, Finland, and former Yugoslavia, in that order (Fig. 3). The Serbian part of the SCS showed similar trends in all-

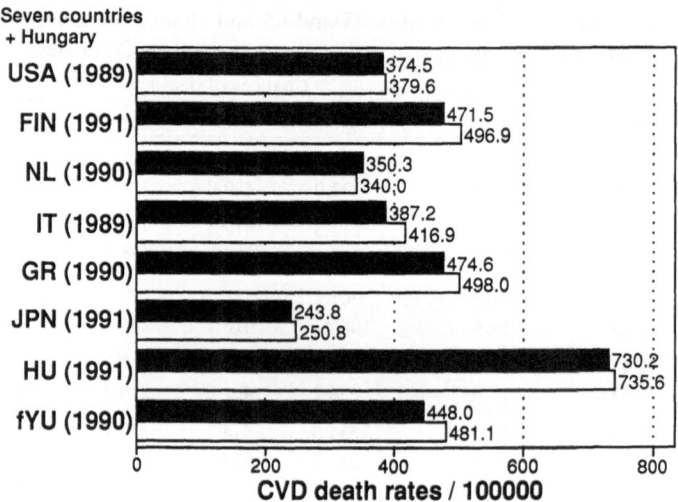

Fig. 3. Cardiovascular mortality for men (*solid bars*) and women (*open bars*) of all ages per 100 000 population in the Seven Countries plus Hungary. (From [3], with permission)

cause and cardiovascular deaths in the cohort of 516 men from Vojvodina followed for 25 years. The data for the whole province of Vojvodina are also comparable with those for Hungary. Overall CVD mortality is higher in women due to their longevity and the chance for developing CVD at ages over 80.

Stroke is the leading cause of cardiovascular mortality in Hungary, Greece, and Italy, and congestive cardiomyopathy in Yugoslavia (Table 3).

U.S. cardiovascular death rates have fallen below those of all European countries participating in the SCS except for the Netherlands; in 1989 for men, 374.5 per 100 000 and for women 379.6, lower than for Greece (men 474.6; women 498.0). (Fig. 3, Table 3). There are limitations of WHO reporting because of variable diagnostic habits in different countries, but the data provide a convenient orientation.

Sex and Age-specific Acute Myocardial Infarction Mortality in fYU and the Seven Countries Plus Hungary

The lowest rates of acute myocardial infarction (AMI) deaths are in Japan, fYU, and Italy (Table 4). The highest rates, (starting at an early age, 35–44), are reported in Finland, followed by Hungary, the Netherlands, and the United States. Acute myocardial infarction deaths are most frequent at ages 65–74 and ≥75 years. At age ≥75 years, AMI death rates in women are also high.

Table 3. All causes and specific CVD mortality, all ages, death rates per 100 000 population Seven Countries + Hungary.

Country	Sex	All causes	All CVD	ARF	RHD	HD	AMI	IHD	CHF + CM	Stroke	Athero sclerosis	PAD	VD	Other CVD
United States 1989	M	921.0	374.5	0.0	1.5	11.3	111.0	101.9	81.8	47.4	6.0	11.9	0.7	1.0
	F	814.3	379.6	0.0	3.3	14.5	88.5	105.5	84.5	69.3	9.5	7.7	0.8	0.9
Finland 1991	M	1009.6	471.5	0.0	1.1	5.8	197.2	101.0	46.8	94.8	7.1	16.2	1.4	0.2
	F	958.7	496.9	0.0	2.5	10.5	166.3	86.4	61.7	145.3	12.9	7.6	3.4	0.3
Netherlands 1990	M	901.7	350.3	0.0	0.2	3.8	135.4	40.6	73.4	66.7	9.7	19.1	0.8	0.7
	F	822.4	340.3	0.0	0.5	6.7	96.5	27.7	89.7	98.7	9.3	9.3	1.2	0.7
Italy 1989	M	993.1	387.2	0.0	2.3	18.7	89.2	54.3	81.9	111.0	17.2	10.4	1.1	1.1
	F	859.4	416.9	0.1	4.3	31.9	51.7	51.4	104.9	139.5	25.5	4.9	1.8	1.0
Greece 1990	M	995.0	474.6	0.0	0.1	9.0	108.1	44.5	150.7	151.3	1.9	7.2	0.1	1.6
	F	873.3	498.0	0.0	0.4	11.3	57.9	30.5	179.9	210.0	3.1	2.5	0.1	2.1
Japan 1991	M	745.3	243.8	0.0	0.7	5.6	29.3	15.8	92.6	92.2	1.4	5.4	0.1	0.6
	F	605.4	250.8	0.0	1.5	9.1	22.6	16.1	95.9	100.0	1.9	3.4	0.1	0.3
f.Yugoslavia 1990	M	957.8	448.0	0.0	1.6	16.5	89.4	12.1	184.4	118.6	21.9	3.1	0.3	0.0
	F	825.1	481.1	0.0	2.1	26.8	48.1	12.1	218.5	139.3	32.0	1.6	0.6	0.0
Hungary 1991	M	1545.6	730.2	0.0	6.1	39.9	174.6	140.3	57.3	190.4	96.1	9.4	15.7	0.4
	F	1265	735.6	0.0	8.7	65.8	109.7	136.3	54.0	215.1	119.1	5.6	20.7	0.6

CVD, cardiovascular disease; ARF, acute rheumatic fever; RHD, rheumatic heart disease; HD, hypertensive disease; AMI, acute myocardial infarction; IHD, ischemic heart disease; CHF, congestive heart failure; CM, cardiomyopathy; PAD, peripheral arterial disease; VD, venous disease. Data from [3].

Table 4. Sex–age specific death rates from acute myocardial infarction per 100 000 population, Seven Countries + Hungary.

Country	Sex	All ages	0	1–4	5–14	15–24	25–34	35–44	45–54	55–64	65–74	≥75 years
United States	M	111.0	0.5	—	—	0.3	2.2	17.1	77.5	225.1	497.1	1278.4
1989	F	88.5	0.4	—	—	0.1	0.7	3.9	20.7	82.7	242.4	910.3
Finland	M	197.2	—	—	—	—	1.5	23.0	101.4	376.7	976.3	2260.7
1991	F	166.3	—	—	—	—	1.1	2.4	12.4	68.8	377.4	1591.5
Netherlands	M	135.4	—	—	—	0.3	2.3	19.0	77.8	256.1	642.9	1503.4
1990	F	96.5	1.0	—	—	0.0	1.1	3.8	16.9	63.8	239.8	962.9
Italy	M	89.2	—	—	—	0.4	3.1	16.3	59.7	173.7	356.4	722.9
1989	F	51.7	—	—	0.0	0.1	0.5	2.4	9.8	36.0	136.2	435.9
Greece	M	108.1	—	—	—	0.5	5.5	30.2	79.4	198.9	403.8	768.5
1990	F	57.9	—	—	—	0.3	1.1	2.4	10.9	43.2	169.7	501.2
Japan	M	29.3	—	—	0.0	0.1	1.0	4.0	14.0	45.9	114.5	355.2
1991	F	22.6	0.3	—	0.0	0.1	0.2	0.9	3.5	13.7	55.5	249.3
f.Yugoslavia	M	89.4	—	—	—	0.9	6.1	31.6	115.4	279.1	465.0	635.4
1990	F	48.1	—	—	—	0.5	2.1	7.2	28.1	92.8	212.9	393.5
Hungary	M	174.6	—	—	—	0.6	15.3	66.4	179.8	429.7	743.2	1120.5
1991	F	109.7	—	—	—	0.4	2.9	15.7	39.3	132.5	352.4	792.8

Data from [3].

Proportional Cardiovascular Versus All-cause Mortality in RYU and Its Republics and Provinces, 1987–1992

In the RYU and its regions cardiovascular deaths contribute 50% of all deaths in men and around 60% in women (Fig. 4). Percentages are higher in Vojvodina for both sexes, reaching as high as 66% in women. The contribution of CVD deaths to all-cause deaths increases with age, reaching more than 70% at ages over 75 years, and is higher in women than in men after age 45.

Trends in CVD Mortality in Serbia and Its provinces and Regions

Linear trend analysis of cardiovascular (WHO *International Classification of Diseases*, code 390–459) mortality during the period 1980–1990 in Serbia (Fig. 5) showed a slight decline [$y = 577 - 2.1x$, with $r = -0.4$, (x, year interval; r, regression coefficient; y, predicted rate per year interval)]. However, regional differences were observed, with decreasing rates in a large Belgrade area, but further increases in Vojvodina, eastern Serbia, and Kosmet [4].

In fYU from 1980–1990, many epidemiological and preventive studies and developments occurred in a number of specialized institutions for prevention and rehabilitation of CVD: in Opatija and Krapinske Toplice (Croatia), in Radenci (Slovenia), in Igalo (Montenegro), and in Niska Banja (Serbia). These interventions probably had an impact on CVD control in fYU and its republics up until 1990.

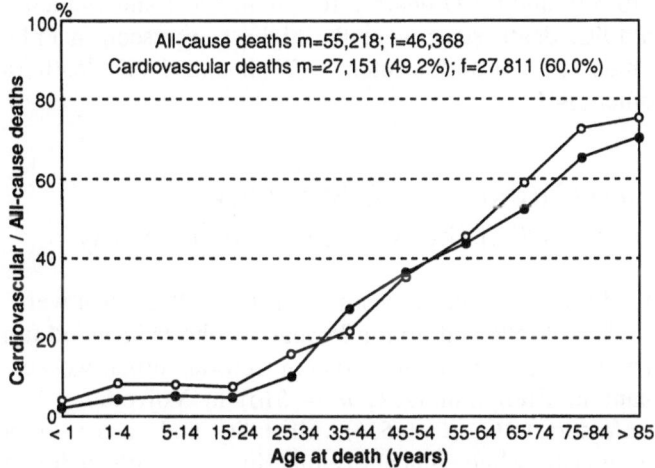

Fig. 4. Sex- and age-specific cardiovascular deaths versus all-cause deaths in women (*open circles*) and men (*closed circles*) in the Republic of Yugoslavia in 1991. *m*, male; *f*, female

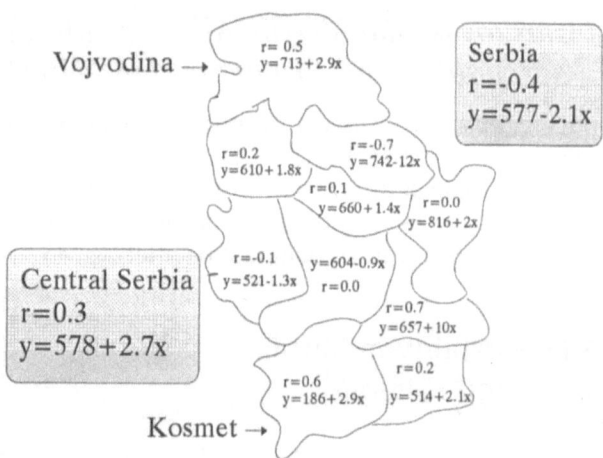

Fig. 5. Cardiovascular mortality trends (WHO IX classification 390–459) in Serbia and its regions, 1980–1990. r, Regression coefficient; y, predicted mortality rate per year; x, year interval. (From [4], with permission)

All-cause and CVD Mortality in Serbia, 1990–1992

It is difficult to judge all the serious consequences on national health of the tragic civil war which broke out in 1991 and is still lingering in some fYU territories. Data on deaths in Central Serbia and Vojvodina (territories of fYU spared by direct war clashes) show dramatic increases in all-cause and CVD death rates, reaching very high values in 1992 for Central Serbia and Vojvodina (Table 5). For Central Serbia, all-cause death rates in 1992 were: men, 1235.3 and women, 1024.9, and CVD death rates: men, 624.1 and women, 629.4. For Vojvodina in 1992, death rates were the highest ever seen in fYU: all-cause death rates: men, 1512.0 and women, 1275.0, and CVD death rates: men, 821.4 and women, 844.5.

All-cause and Cardiovascular Mortality in the Serbian Part of the Seven Countries Study

Three cohorts of men aged 40–59 years at entry in 1962–1964 were studied as a part of the SCS and followed up for 25 years. Cohorts included farmers from the village of Velika Krsna (VK, $n = 511$) in Central Serbia, workers of a food processing plant in Zrenjanin (ZR, $n = 516$) in Vojvodina, and Belgrade University professors (BG, $n = 536$). Mortality and causes of death were followed continuously, while clinical examinations and surveys for the classical risk factors of CVD were repeated at intervals of 5 years. Most of the findings from the three Serbian cohorts were analyzed centrally in Minneapolis and Rome, exploiting the data base of all 16 cohorts. Studies of cohort differences

Table 5. All-cause and specific CVD deaths, all ages, per 100 000 population, Central Serbia and Vojvodina, 1990–1992.

Region	Year	Sex	All causes	All CVD	RHD	HD	IHD	AMI	CHF CM	Stroke	Other CVD
Central	1990	M	1115.5	559.6	1.2	25.4	104.9	included	262.9	145.6	20.4
Serbia		F	947.9	576.3	1.3	39.8	59.1	in IHD	285.8	163.1	27.2
	1991	M	1174.0	577.0	1.7	28.6	118.7	included	250.6	154.7	22.4
		F	981.0	587.0	2.4	45.3	66.2	in IHD	272.8	175.0	25.6
	1992	M	1235.3	624.1	3.0	39.1	37.6	193.5	429.9	235.0	36.7
		F	1024.9	629.4	4.4	61.4	20.1	98.1	490.8	256.9	47.5
Vojvodina	1990	M	1333.1	720.2	3.4	10.4	172.5	included	301.8	175.2	56.8
		F	1134.7	744.5	3.9	16.6	93.0	in IHD	356.5	191.1	83.5
	1991	M	1447.0	769.0	3.2	13.0	191.0	included	317.2	188.6	56.1
		F	1197.0	794.0	3.0	19.7	103.1	in IHD	371.5	206.9	89.7
	1992	M	1512.0	821.4	4.5	14.0	6.2	202.1	346.7	191.4	56.5
		F	1275.0	844.5	2.9	21.8	7.2	106.2	419.0	204.9	82.7

CVD, cardiovascular disease; RHD, rheumatic heart disease; HD, hypertensive disease; AMI, acute myocardial infarction; IHD, ischemic heart disease; CHF, congestive heart disease; CM, cardiomyopathy.
Data from [10].

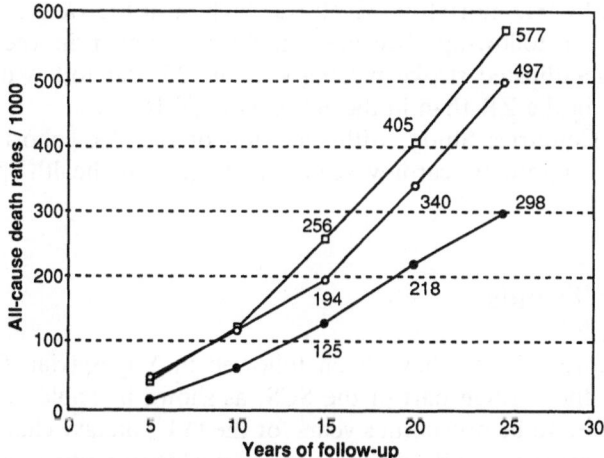

Fig. 6. Serbia—Seven Countries Study. Age-adjusted all-cause mortality in men aged 40–59 at entry. *Open squares*, Zrenjanin; *open circles*, Krsna; *closed circles*, Belgrade

in prevalence and incidence of CVD and coronary heart disease are still in progress [9,11–15].

The three Serbian cohorts showed the lowest prevalence of CVD at the beginning of the SCS, along with Japanese, Italian, and Greek cohorts. This trend lasted for the first 5 to 10 years of follow-up. However, after 15 to 25 years of follow-up, age-adjusted rates for all causes (Fig. 6) and specific causes

Table 6. Age-adjusted death rates per 1000 population from specific causes in 25 years in three Serbian cohorts.

	Cohort		
	VK	ZR	BG
CHD	122	177	118
Stroke	93	120	45
Cancer	103	130	85
Other	179	150	50
All causes	497	577	298

CHD, coronary heart disease; VK, Velika Krsna; ZR, Zrenjanin; BG, Beograd.
Data from [14].

(coronary heart disease, stroke, all CVD, and cancer) were significantly higher in the ZR cohort (Table 6). BG professors enjoyed an exceedingly better survival at follow-ups of 15, 20, and 25 years [13,14].

Age-adjusted CHD mortality, which was highest in the Belgrade professors until the 10-year follow-up, became significantly higher in the ZR cohort thereafter. Age-adjusted stroke mortality at the 25-year follow-up was significantly higher in the ZR than in the BG cohort (Table 6).

The Seven Countries Study, with inclusion of the ZR cohort since 1963, indicates the important cardiovascular and general health problems in Vojvodina.

Risk-factor Trends

Selected CVD risk factors have been followed in Yugoslavian CVD studies [16,17] and in the Serbian part of the SCS, as shown in Table 7. In the early 1970s, considered to be prosperous years for the fYU, dietary changes included higher consumption of total energy, and greater consumption of animal fats at the expense of carbohydrates. Dietary habits in the fYU in 1964 were estimated by the food consumption method, applied to 150 families examined in the SCS [5–7].

Food consumption patterns have been changing since the 1960s in all of the Seven Countries [18], showing increased consumption of meat, eggs, dairy products, fats and oils, and desserts in the Mediterranean countries. These changes correspond to the fYU trends found in consumption of foods from 1952 to 1987.

In contrast to most cohorts of the SCS, Serbian cohorts showed dramatic increases in mean cholesterol level during the first 10 years of follow-up: for

Table 7. Mean levels of selected risk factors in men free from major CHD events at years 0, 5, and 10.

Factors	Mean levels		
	Year 0	Year 5	Year 10
Velika Krsna	$n = 504$	$n = 457$	$n = 432$
Age (years)	49.9 ± 6.6	54.6 ± 6.2	59.4 ± 6.1
Body mass index (kg/m²)	22.0 ± 2.6	22.4 ± 3.1	22.4 ± 3.3
Cigarettes (n/day)	8.0 ± 9.6	7.8 ± 10.1	7.3 ± 9.8
Systolic blood pressure (mm Hg)	131.4 ± 18.5	129.7 ± 18.3	144.1 ± 22.4
Serum cholesterol (mg/dl)	159.9 ± 31.3	171.7 ± 35.0	190.2 ± 36.5
Zrenjanin	$n = 508$	$n = 469$	$n = 428$
Age (years)	49.1 ± 5.4	54.1 ± 5.4	58.8 ± 5.3
Body mass index (kg/m²)	25.1 ± 3.6	26.2 ± 4.0	26.3 ± 4.1
Cigarettes (n/day)	11.8 ± 11.5	14.1 ± 13.2	12.5 ± 13.5
Systolic blood pressure (mm Hg)	133.5 ± 18.7	144.2 ± 23.7	149.0 ± 25.5
Serum cholesterol (mg/dl)	168.7 ± 32.6	207.2 ± 38.9	230.4 ± 45.8
Beograd	$n = 530$	$n = 440$	$n = 409$
Age (years)	47.7 ± 5.6	52.7 ± 5.6	57.7 ± 5.7
Body mass index (kg/m²)	26.2 ± 2.9	26.8 ± 2.8	26.5 ± 2.9
Cigarettes (n/day)	10.2 ± 14.0	9.6 ± 14.6	7.6 ± 13.6
Systolic blood pressure (mm Hg)	133.8 ± 18.0	135.6 ± 20.4	144.0 ± 21.4
Serum cholesterol (mg/dl)	210.2 ± 41.0	243.2 ± 44.8	246.2 ± 43.3

Data from [14].

ZR, 36.5%; for VK, 18.5%; and for BG, 15.3%. In the other 13 SCS cohorts, serum cholesterolemia increased far less over time [9,14,15].

Discussion

Political events occurring in the 3 years since 1990 led, at the beginning of 1992, to the breakup of the fYU into new states: Slovenia, Croatia, Bosnia and Herzegovina; the former republic of Macedonia; and the Federal Republic of Yugoslavia (Serbia plus Montenegro). Lingering civil war in some fYU territories has brought about a disaster, with many lives lost and people struggling for elementary existence. There are more than 2 million displaced persons, of which around 700 000 are in Serbia and Montenegro, depending on humanitarian aid.

Those events have adversely influenced, in a relatively short time, the general level of health, leading to sharp increases of all-cause and CVD deaths. Health services and research in medicine are severely jeopardized because of economic depression in the RYU and broken ties within the fYU and with the international community.

This paper includes a limited presentation and comments on cardiovascular diseases in Yugoslavia based on recent data prepared by the Federal Institute of Statistics and by the Federal Public Health Department, and respective services of the republics of Serbia and Montenegro.

Former Yugoslavia was active among 168 other states in the WHO program, "Health for All in the Year 2000," and regularly reported data on 12 global indicators on human health. The 1992 *World Health Statistics Annual*, published in 1993 [3], has been used for comparison of cardiovascular death rates in the fYU and other countries participating in the SCS. Hungary was included in the comparisons because in the late 1960s, Ancel Keys was planning to include Hungarian cardiovascular field surveys in the region of Segedin, to make the Seven Countries Study an Eight Countries Study. The other obvious reason is the close similarity in general health and cardiovascular pathology and in dietary and lifestyle habits between Hungary and Slavonia, Vojvodina, and Serbia.

Demographic changes in the fYU in the last 50 years have been characterized by a steady increase in absolute numbers of inhabitants, but with a relatively larger decline in live births, the growth rate approaching only 0.3 per 100 in 1990. In the northern Serbian province of Vojvodina in the last 5 years, mortality rates overtook birth rates in the proportion of 12.3 to 11.2 per 1000. From 1950 until 1990, former Yugoslavs had reached an average life expectancy of around 69 years for men and 75 years for women. However, compared with life expectancy for Japanese and populations in other countries in which the SCS was carried out, fYU life expectancy estimates were lower.

Comparing data for the Seven Countries and Hungary, it can be seen that CVD death rates for the fYU in 1990 reached rates of 448 for men and 481 for women, lower than in Greece, Finland, and Hungary. However, Hungary, with very high CVD mortality rates in 1991 (men 730 and women 736) could be compared to Vojvodina, the northern province of Serbia, in which CVD mortality rates were high in 1991 (men 769 and women 794), and in 1992 even higher.

AMI mortality in the fYU in 1990 was among the lowest in all the Seven Countries or Hungary. According to data from 1992 for Central Serbia and Vojvodina, however, rates are now well over the rates reported for the other areas, reaching in Vojvodina 202 for men and 106 for women.

CVD deaths have dramatically changed in fYU over a few decades, first with an upward trend until 1980, reaching rates at the level of developed countries, then with a stable line and even slight decline until 1990, but in the last two years, 1991–1992, experiencing a new dramatic jump in rates in Vojvodina and Central Serbia.

CVD mortality contributes proportionately more than 50% in men and more than 60% in women to all-cause mortality. Zrenjanin cohort has been at the highest risk of CVD and all-cause deaths, representative of the situation in the whole of Vojvodina.

The survival of Belgrade University professors was the most favorable of all cohorts in the SCS except for Crete, with 25-year follow-up rates for CVD at 198 (per 1000) and for all-cause deaths, at 347 (per 1000). The cohort of Velika

Krsna was in between, but there most CVD deaths were from pulmonary heart disease as a consequence of tuberculosis and chronic bronchitis.

Serbian cohorts have been characterized by excessive increases in serum cholesterol level in the first 10 years of follow-up, significantly more than in other SCS cohorts. Those changes were most intensive in the ZR cohort (Vojvodina), due more to real trends than to aging.

Changes over time in dietary habits in the fYU have also been great, with greater intake of total energy and more consumption of saturated fats and dietary cholesterol at the expense of carbohydrates. However, from 1990 until 1993, and at present, food shortages have significantly influenced the dietary habits of the general population in the fYU territories and the RYU.

Acknowledgments. I am sincerely grateful to the hosts and chairman of this meeting, the honorable Professor Hironori Toshima, and coeditors of the proceedings, Ancel Keys and Henry Blackburn, founders of the SCS, for affording me the great opportunity to participate, present, and submit this paper from the Symposium "Lessons for Science from the Seven Countries Study," held in Fukuoka, Japan.

References

1. Demografska statistika 1990 (1992) Federal Institute of Statistics, Belgrade, pp 1–277
2. Statisticki godisnjak '91 (1992) Federal Institute of Public Health, Belgrade, pp 1–158
3. 1992 World health statistics annual (1993) World Health Organization, Geneva, Sect. C, pp C3–C13, Sect. D, pp D107–D332
4. Djordjevic M, Mitrovic N, Vuletic Z, Markovic Lj, Breznik D, Andjelic N (1993) Demographic trends and health status in Serbia and Kosovo Metohija. Jugoslavija Publik, Beograd, pp 1–242
5. Djordjevic B, Simic B, Simic A, Strasser T, Josipovic V, Macarol V, Klinc I, Nedeljkovic S, Todorovic P (1965) Dietary studies in connection with epidemiology of heart diseases: results in Serbia. Voeding 26:117–127
6. Djordjevic SB, Josipovic V, Nedeljkovic IS, Strasser T, Slavkovic V, Simic B, Keys A, Blackburn H (1966) Men in Velika Krsna, a Serbian village. In: Keys A, Aravanis C, Blackburn H, van Buchem FSP, Buzina R, Djordjevic SB, Dontas SA, Fidanza F, Karvonen JM, Kimura M, Lekos D, Monti M, Puddu V, Taylor HL (eds), Epidemiological studies related to coronary heart disease. Characteristics of men aged 40–59 in Seven Countries. Acta Med Scand, Tampere 1967 [Suppl 460]:267–277
7. Djordjevic B, Balog B, Bozinovic LJ, Josipovic V, Nedeljkovic S, Lambic I, Sekulic S, Slavkovic V, Stojanovic G, Simic A, Simic B, Strasser T, Blackburn H, Keys A (1970) Three cohorts of men followed five years in Serbia. In: Keys A (ed), Coronary heart disease in seven countries. American Heart Association Monograph No. 29. American Heart Association, New York, pp I-123, I-137

 8. Keys A, Menotti A, Aravanis C, Blackburn H, Djordjevic B, Buzina R, Dontas A, Fidanza F, Karvonen M, Kimura N, Mohacek I, Nedeljkovic S, Puddu V, Punsar S, Taylor H, Conti S, Kromhout D, Toshima H (1984) The Seven Countries Study: 2,289 deaths in 15 years. Prev Med 13:141–154
 9. Keys A, Aravanis C, Blackburn H, Buzina R, Djordjevic B, Dontas A, Fidanza F, Karvonen M, Kimura N, Menotti A, Mohacek I, Nedeljkovic S, Puddu V, Punsar S, Taylor H, van Buchem FSP (1980) Seven Countries Study. A multivariate analysis of death and coronary heart disease. Harvard University Press, Cambridge, Mass., pp 1–381
10. Demografska statistika (1993) Federal Institute of Statistics, Belgrade
11. Keys A, Menotti A, Karvonen M, Aravanis C, Blackburn H, Buzina R, Djordjevic B, Dontas A, Fidanza F, Keys M, Kromhout D, Nedeljkovic S, Punsar S, Seccareccia F, Toshima H (1986) The diet and 15-year death rates in the Seven Countries Study. Am J Epidemiol 124(6):903–915
12. Menotti A, Keys A, Aravanis C, Blackburn H, Dontas A, Fidanza F, Karvonen JM, Kromhout D, Nedeljkovic S, Nissinen A, Pekkarinen J, Toshima H (1989) Seven Countries Study. First 20 year mortality data in 12 cohorts of six countries. Ann Med 21:175–179
13. Nedeljkovic S, Menotti A, Keys A, Ostojic M, Grujic M, Kromhout D, Stojanovic G (1992) Coronary heart disease in three cohorts of men in Serbia followed-up for 25 years as a part of the Seven Countries Study. Kardiologija 13:35–44
14. Nedeljkovic S, Ostojic M, Grujic M, Josipovic V, Keys A, Menotti A, Seccareccia F, Lanti M, Kromhout D (1993) Coronary heart disease deaths in 25 years. The experience in the three Serbian cohorts of the Seven Countries Study. Acta Cardiol 48:11–24
15. Menotti A, Keys A, Kromhout D, Blackburn H, Aravanis C, Bleomberg B, Buzina R, Dontas A, Fidanza F, Giampaoli S, Karvonen JM, Lanti M, Mohacek I, Nedeljkovic S, Nissinen A, Pekkanen J, Punsar S, Seccareccia F, Toshima H (1993) Intercohort differences in coronary heart disease mortality in the 25-year follow-up of the Seven Countries Study. Eur J Epidemiol 9(5):527–536
16. Kozarevic D, Pirc B, Vojvodic N, Dawber TR, Gordon T, Zukel WJ (1977) The Yugoslavia Cardiovascular Study. III—Deaths by case and area. Int J Epidemiol 6:129–134
17. Vukotic M, Nedeljkovic S, Mujovic V, Djukic V (1991) Cardiovascular diseases. Epidemiology and prevention. Rakovica Cardiovascular Study (RASCO), Medical Faculty of Belgrade edition, Beograd, pp 1–80
18. Kromhout D, Keys A, Aravanis C, Buzina R, Fidanza F, Giampaoli S, Jansen A, Menotti A, Nedeljkovic S, Pekkarinen J, Simic SB, Toshima H (1989) Food consumption patterns in the 1960s in seven countries. Am J Clin Nutr 49:889–894

Discussion

Asian-Pacific seminar student: Concerning cardiovascular mortality in women, have you divided the population into pre- and postmenopausal?

S. Nedeljkovic: Much is related to the reproductive status of women. After menopause there is an increase in rates to exceed those of men. Moreover, bypass therapy poses a greater risk in women. These are among problems we should address in the future.

Same student: In our country, India, if we look at age-specific data, we find large differences between men and women. Maybe combining these data is giving us an inaccurate picture.

H. Ueshima: I understand your conclusion that the increase in coronary disease may be attributed to the increase in average cholesterol level. How about other risk factors? What are the trends in smoking and hypertension?

S. Nedeljkovic: I forgot to say that dietary changes have been very large in Yugoslavia over the last 3 to 4 decades. Thoroughgoing, definitive dietary studies in individual subjects have been accumulated in all Yugoslavian cohorts of the Seven Countries Study. In Vojvodina, for example, daily consumption of fats is now about 150 g compared to Japan, where you now have about 50 g. So I am rather convinced of the basic idea of Ancel Keys, that dietary fat and cholesterol must be the major risk factors responsible for population differences in blood lipids and probably in coronary disease.

Related to this issue are Kromhout's studies in The Netherlands among surviving members of the Seven Countries cohort which show that serum cholesterol levels there are quite stable. Moreover, body weight is practically unchanging in that cohort. Blood pressure, however, is increasing as the cohort ages.

Recent Trends in Cardiovascular Disease and Risk Factors in the Seven Countries Study: Greece

ANASTASIOS S. DONTAS

Summary. In the past 30 years, Greece has experienced marked but uneven socioeconomic development, with average income increasing about 20-fold. Consequently, the lifestyle of people throughout the country has changed dramatically. Stable, age-old dietary habits and high habitual physical activity have gradually given way to "Western"-type diets and a more sedentary lifestyle. Smoking has become an almost universal habit which only very recently has shown signs of leveling off. As a result, body mass index, blood pressure, cholesterol levels, and frequency of diabetes mellitus have increased by varying degrees, particularly in urban areas and those prominently affected by tourism. Simultaneously, mortality rates from coronary heart disease, other heart diseases, malignant neoplasms (cancer of the lung), diabetes, and traffic accidents have markedly increased at the national level. Nevertheless, several aspects of the traditional Greek way of life and diet—notably, a relatively high consumption of vegetables and fruits, olive oil, and bread—remain entrenched among large segments of the Greek population. This may explain why a population with few healthy habits and an imperfect health system today still enjoys one of the longer life expectancies in the world.

Key words. Cardiovascular disease risk factors—Diet—Cholesterol—Physical activity—Smoking—Greece

Introduction

Of the 16 cohorts in the Seven Countries Study, those of Crete (686 men) and Corfu (529 men) have developed the lowest rates of coronary heart disease (CHD) mortality as well as mortality from all causes in 10 and 20 years of follow-up [1–3] (Table 1). The areas of the Seven Countries examined, however, varied not only with respect to diet, physical activity, and climate, but also in socioeconomic status. For example, the cohorts of Greece, Italy, and provinces of former Yugoslavia had a lower socioeconomic level than those of the Netherlands, Finland, or the United States.

Table 1. Twenty-year standardized death rates per 1000 population from all causes (ALL) and coronary heart disease (CHD).

Cohort	ALL Rate	ALL 95% CL	CHD Rate	CHD 95% CL	CHD/ALL (%[a])
EF-SF	469	436–501	236	208–264	48.7
WF-SF	393	361–425	151	127–175	38.4
ZU-NL	319	289–349	122	100–144	38.2
CV-IT	375	346–404	93	75–111	24.8
MO-IT	322	290–354	75	56–94	23.3
RR-IT	263	233–293	82	63–101	31.2
VK-YU	316	278–354	61	40–82	19.3
ZR-YU	390	349–431	97	72–122	24.9
CT-GR	172	145–199	13	5–21	7.6
CO-GR	239	203–274	39	23–55	16.3
TA-JAP	286	248–324	26	11–41	9.1
UH-JAP	366	325–407	34	18–50	9.3

EF-SF, East Finland; WF, SF West Finland; ZU-NL, Zutphen, Netherlands; CV-IT, Crevalcore, Italy; MO-IT, Montegiorgio, Italy; RR-IT, Railroad sample, Italy; VK-YU, Velika Krsna, Yugoslavia; ZR-YU, Zrenjanin, Yugoslavia; CT-GR, Crete, Greece; CO-GR, Corfu, Greece; TA-JAP, Tanushimaru, Japan; UH-JAP, Ushibuka, Japan; CL, confidence limits.
[a] Proportion of CHD on ALL.
Data from [3].

This chapter presents the current health status of the Greek population and recent trends in total cardiovascular disease mortality. Furthermore, it evaluates risk-factor changes in the original Cretan cohort examined in 1960 as well as in other Greek cohorts examined and followed up since the 1960s. The original Corfu cohort, initially investigated in 1961, has been less easily followed, and data on risk-factor changes of this sample are not available beyond the 5- and 10-year resurveys.

Evaluation of the health status of the country as a whole has been based on demographic data, on total and cause-specific mortality rates in Greece and other European countries, and on potential years of life lost. Age standardization was computed from the European standard population.

The Greek Economy–Health Services

Table 2 presents the main characteristics of the Greek economy and society in 1989 [4]. It indicates the relatively high economic inflation rate, which remains today (1993), more than three times higher than the average of the 11 other European Community (EC) member states.

Table 2. Characteristics of the Greek economy and society in 1989.

GNP/person	U.S. $4 087
Inflation rate	15.5%
Unemployment rate/working force	7.5%
Social expenditures	24.4% GNP
Public expenditures for health	5.2% GNP
Private expenditures for health	3.1% GNP
Life expectancy	
At birth	Men: 74 years Women: 79 years
At age 65	Men: 15.2 years Women 17.7 years
Infant mortality	10 per 1000 births

GNP, gross national product.
Data from [4].

The yearly increase in expenditures on health and social security (particularly in the public sector) exceeds the rate of growth in the gross national product (GNP). This is thought to be related to:

a) The rapid growth of the aged segment of the population: subjects aged ≥65 years presently make up more than 14% of the population and increase by 1% per decade. Greece also has a very rapid increase of subjects aged ≥80 years, presently 389 200 and expected to reach 468 600 by the year 2000 (i.e., from 3.91% to 4.73% of the population), who are high consumers of health services.

b) The altered spectrum of diseases and the emergence of chronic and debilitating, slowly fatal diseases that require high-cost techniques for diagnosis, therapy, and long-term care.

c) Improved socioeconomic status and public information resulting in increased demand for and use of health services.

d) Health providers costs increasing faster than the GNP.

The composition of health care expenditures by the public and private sectors is diametrically different, indicating the opposing orientation in health care targets, as well as the efforts by the state to acquire and control all hospital medical centers. In 1991 *public* expenditures for health were 63.5% for hospital costs, 15.8% for drug costs, and 12.5% for nonhospital care. *Private* expenditures were 67.5% for nonhospital care, 16.4% for drug costs, and 16% for hospital care.

Ideologically, there has been a significant shift in the past 20 years in the philosophy underlying health service in Greece. Until the late 1970s, the prevailing view of health care stressed treatment rather than prevention, had the doctor as the pivot of the system, and supported a mixture of private medicine for those who could afford to pay and public medicine for those who could not. In hospital health care, there were three classes of public beds, reflecting the benefit level of the various insurance funds or supplementary payments.

The introduction of the National Health System in 1983 marked an attempt to change the doctor-centered idea of health care to a more comprehensive and egalitarian system for patients and toward decentralized health services. This latter, evidenced in the setting up of university hospitals in several capitals of the major regions, was a policy initiated in the late 1970s which has continued at a rapid pace until today (1993).

Physicians

The number of physicians has increased at an accelerating pace during the past 30 years. Greece presently has one of the highest proportions of physicians for its population (1:289 population). Physician services are, however, not evenly distributed; it is estimated that 70% of physicians are concentrated in the regions of Athens and Thessaloniki where about 40% of the population lives. In contrast, areas such as the Ionian Islands (Corfu) and the island of Evoia near Athens have a physician to population ratio of 1:1009 and 1:1330, respectively.

Nurses

Historically, nursing has had a low standard and been numerically inadequate (1:462 population). Even in major hospitals, "nursing care" is still largely provided by patients families or privately paid personnel, often an essential supplement to inadequate or indifferent staff nursing services. This is particularly a problem for the sick and disabled elderly who may be hospitalized for long periods, putting a heavy burden on the family and leading to inadequate care for the isolated elderly.

The centralization of higher education for nurses (3–4 years post high school), and the establishment since 1980 of a university nursing school of 4 years training, have aimed at increasing the numbers and upgrading the social and professional status of registered nurses, possibly at the cost of practical knowledge and experience. Tangible effects of recent efforts to reduce the disparity between the high density of physicians and the low density of nursing personnel will take some years to appear.

Health Services

Health services are distributed through public and private sectors, despite significant efforts by the government in the early 1980s to diminish the private sector and to ensure an evenly distributed health service system of high quality, accessible to all citizens at their locus of residence, all through the newly established National Health Service. This target has only partially been achieved, because the concentration of health services and the influx of patients to metropolitan centers continue unabated, and because a significant black market in health supplies still flourishes, while the private hospital sector, although reduced in number of beds, has been modernized so that the surviving units are financially flourishing. The total number of beds in 1980 was 59 400, of which 25 900 belonged to the public sector, 25 100 to the private sector, and 8400 to the nonprofit private sector. In 1987 these numbers were: total beds, 51 500; public sector, 35 300; private, 15 900; and nonprofit private, 300.

General Mortality Trends

Age-adjusted total mortality rates in Greece have been gradually declining during the last decades, particularly in women (Fig. 1) [4], so that the level of mortality in 1988 was among the lowest in Europe (756.3 per 100 000 total population; 916.4 in men, 616.9 in women). This generally low mortality is mainly due to the low mortality from coronary heart disease (CHD) and to relatively low rates from certain neoplastic diseases. This exceptional position, however, is gradually receding. Greece dropped from first place in 1970–1974 to second in 1975–1984, behind Iceland. It is expected to recede to third place in 2000.

Life Expectancy

Concurrently with low mortality, the life expectancy of Greeks is among the highest in Europe (for men it is the highest among 24 European countries at ages 0 and 65) (Figs. 2, 3) [4]. The life expectancy for Greek women, although longer by almost 5 years at birth than that of Greek men (78.9 years), is rela-

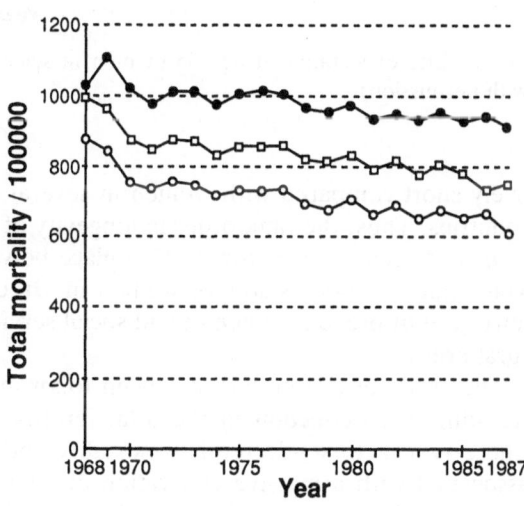

Fig. 1. Age-standardized (European) annual mortality (per 100 000 population) from all causes in Greek men (*closed circles*), women (*open circles*), and total population (*open squares*), 1968–1987. (From [4], with permission)

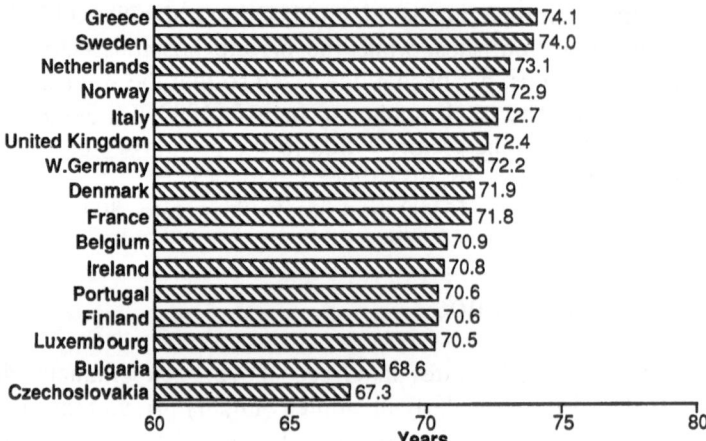

Fig. 2. Life expectancy at birth of men in selected European countries. (From [4], with permission)

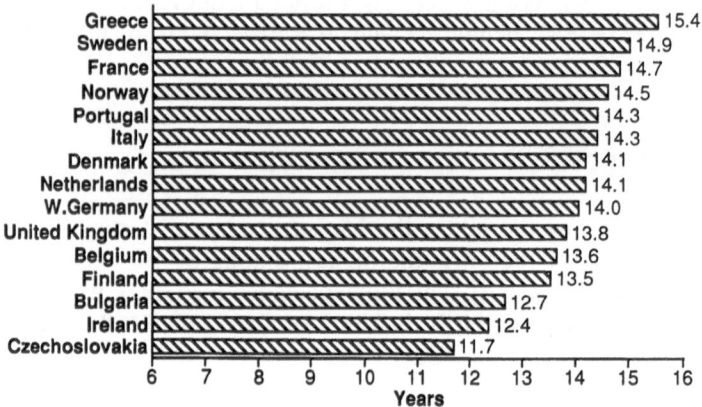

Fig. 3. Life expectancy at age 65 of men in selected European countries. (From [4], with permission)

tively short compared with women in several northern and western European countries. Thus, the rank order in longevity of Greek women among European women decreased from 8th to 11th place between the ages of 0 and 65 years. This relatively poor status of women in Greece is attributed in part to their lower use of preventive health and social services in contrast to men, chiefly in rural areas.

The crude birth rate has also been following a downward trend since 1950, resulting in a reduction in the total fertility rate and net reproduction rate. These two factors—decreasing mortality and decreasing reproduction rate—associated with a massive emigration of young and middle-aged adults in the 1960s, resulted in a sudden and dramatic demographic aging of the Greek population, with important economic and sociomedical consequences. It is expected that in 2000, subjects aged 60 and over will constitute 19.7% of the population and those 75 and over, 4.7% of the population.

Cause-specific Mortality

The current major causes of mortality in the Greek population are diseases of the cardiovascular system (50% of all deaths), malignant neoplasms (21%), accidents (5%), and respiratory diseases (5%). These rates approximate those of other developed countries with important temporal differentiations within each class. For example, mortality from infectious diseases (Fig. 4) [4] markedly decreased in the years 1968–1985, but has leveled off since then. Vascular accidents of the central nervous system (CNS) (Fig. 5) [4] and suicide deaths

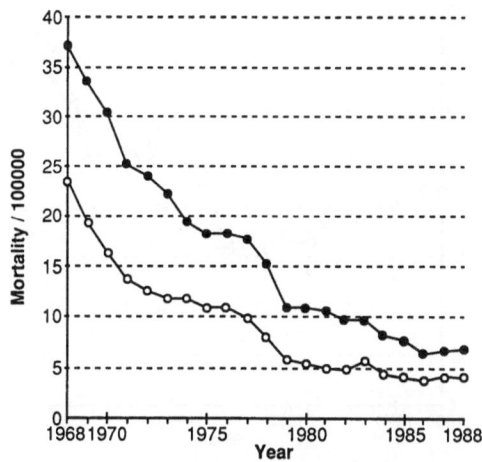

Fig. 4. Age-standardized (European) mortality rates (per 100 000 population) from infectious diseases in Greek men (*closed circles*) and women (*open circles*), 1968–1988. (From [4], with permission)

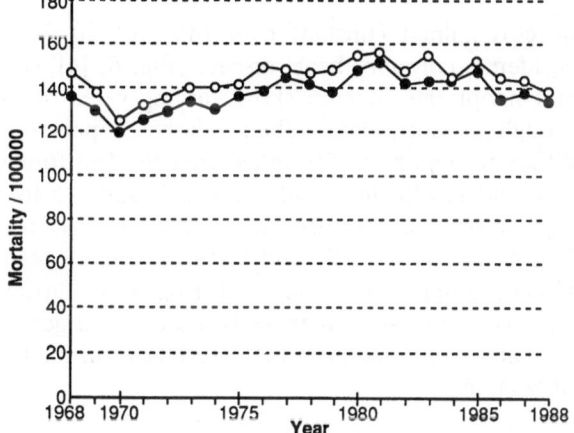

Fig. 5. Age-standardized (European) mortality rates (per 100 000 population) from vascular accidents of the central nervous system in Greek men (*closed circles*) and women (*open circles*), 1968–1988. (From [4], with permission)

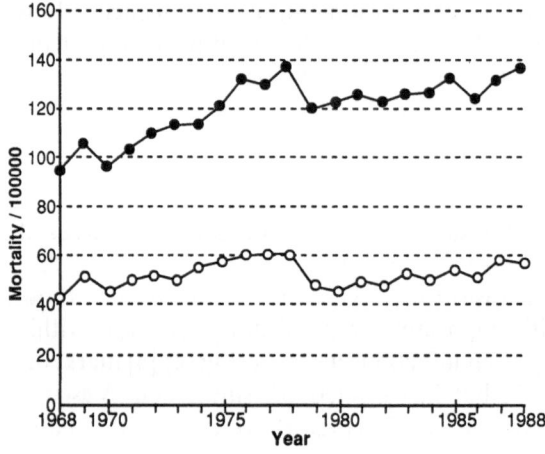

Fig. 6. Age-standardized (European) mortality rates (per 100000 population) for ischemic heart disease in Greek men (*closed circles*) and women (*open circles*), 1968–1988. (From [4], with permission)

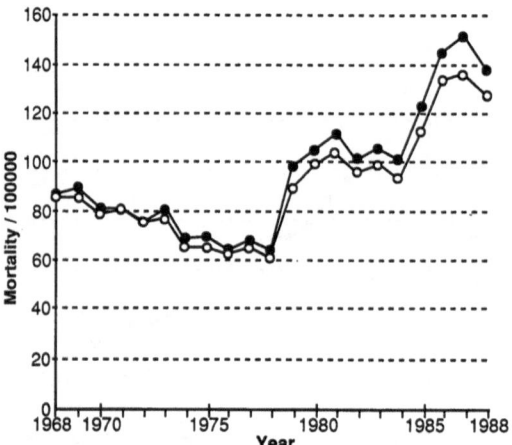

Fig. 7. Age-standardized (European) mortality rates (per 100000 population) for heart diseases other than ischemic in Greek men (*closed circles*) and women (*open circles*), 1968–1988. (From [4], with permission)

have remained constant over the past 20 years. In contrast, deaths from accidents, coronary heart disease (Fig. 6) [4], other heart disease (Fig. 7) [4], and neoplasms in men show varying rates of increase in the last 20 years, though proportionately their relative impact on total mortality is markedly different. The mortality rates from the last four causes in 1988 were 28, 135, 140, and 215 for men and 9, 55, 125, and 115 for women (per 100000). These rates represent increases of 53.2%, 31.7%, 69.6%, and 17% in men and 75.5%, 16.5%, 59.9%, and 6.9% in women, respectively, in the last 20 years. Greece is thus one of the few European countries with an increasing mortality from coronary and other heart diseases. In general, specific mortality rates in men are higher and have increased faster in the last 20 years compared to those of women.

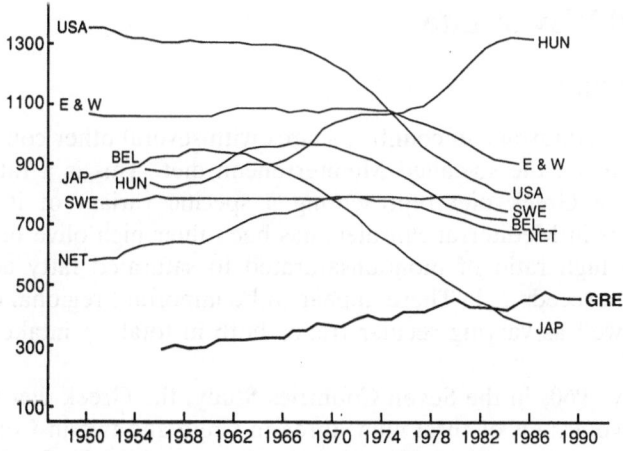

Fig. 8. Trends in mortality of men aged 45–74 years from cardiovascular diseases in the United States; East and West Finland (*E&W*), Hungary (*HUN*), Sweden (*SWE*), Belgium (*BEL*), the Netherlands (*NET*), Greece (*GRE*); and Japan (*JAP*). (Unpublished data)

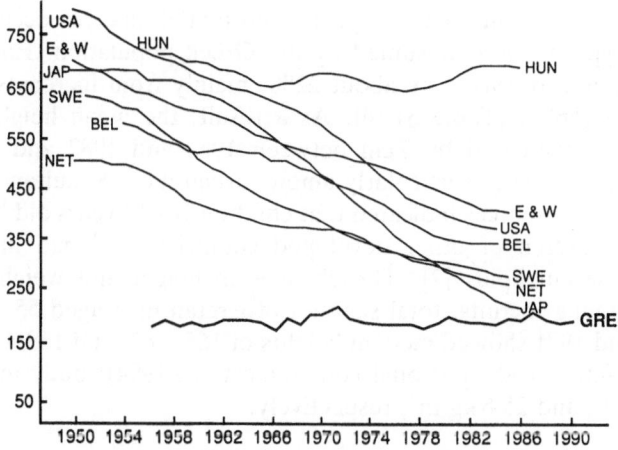

Fig. 9. Trends in mortality of women aged 45–74 years from cardiovascular diseases in the United States; East and West Finland (*E&W*), Hungary (*HUN*), Sweden (*SWE*), Belgium (*BEL*), the Netherlands (*NET*), Greece (*GRE*); and Japan. (Unpublished data)

Figures 8 and 9 show the trends in mortality from cardiovascular diseases in six European countries, the United States, and Japan during the last 35 years. Most countries, led by Japan and the United States, are currently experiencing well-recognized declines in cardiovascular mortality, whereas Greece and particularly Hungary show upward trends, especially in men.

Health and Way of Life

Dietary Habits

Greece, as a Mediterranean country, shares with several other countries lining the Mediterranean the so-called Mediterranean diet. This is a rather loosely used term, the Greek diet representing a specific variant of it. The main common factor in Mediterranean diets has been their high olive oil and bread intake and a high ratio of monounsaturated to saturated fatty acids (M/S), which usually exceeds 2:1. There appear to be important regional differences, however, as well as varying secular trends both in total fat intake and in the ratios of M/S.

In the early 1960s in the Seven Countries Study, the Greek diet was studied in detail in five groups of rural men, three in Crete and two in Corfu, totaling 69 subjects 40–59 years old [5]. Both in Crete and in Corfu the diet was dominated by olive oil, bread, and fruit. These three items alone accounted for 60% or more of total calories; 40.3% of the daily calories in Crete and 32.7% in Corfu were provided by fat, with a ratio between P:S:M fatty acids of roughly 1:2.5:10. About 10.5% and 11.4%, respectively, of calories came from proteins, but only 3%–4% of protein calories were of animal origin.

During the subsequent 25 to 30 years, substantial changes occurred in the amount and type of food consumed by the Greek population. Energy intake during this period increased by about 22%, mainly from increases in protein (19%) and fat (56%) (Table 3) [6]. As a result, the mean height of young military recruits increased by 7 cm between 1968 and 1982 and their mean weight increased by 4 kg, particularly among urban men. Simultaneously, data published in Greek sources indicated that children 10–14 years old had become heavier than children of other developed countries, and had higher blood pressure and serum lipids [7]. The changes in height and weight were not restricted to young recruits; total samples of Cretan men aged 55–59 years in 1960, 1982, and 1991 showed median heights of 165, 167, and 169.4 cm, respectively [8] (Kafatos et al., personal communication, 1994); body mass indexes were 22.6, 26.9, and 25.8 kg/m^2, respectively.

Table 3. Changes in total caloric and specific macro-nutrient intake in Greece over a 20-year period.

	1961–1965	1981–1985	20-Year change
Total daily calories	2990	3650	+22%
Calories from:			
Proteins	361	428	+19%
Fats	841	1312	+56%
Carbohydrates	1708	1793	+5%
Alcoholic drinks	80	117	+46%

Data from [6].

The Cretan food consumption pattern was simple in the 1960s, consisting of whole wheat bread, olive oil, pulses, nuts, vegetables, fruits, and small amounts of milk and cheese. Fish (fresh, salted, or canned) was consumed once a week, and meat was rarely consumed [5,9].

In a 1988 survey of 387 Cretan men and women bank employees living near the area originally studied in 1960, dietary patterns appeared to have markedly changed (Tables 4, 5) [5,10]. A mild decrease in overall caloric intake (from 2685 Kcal/day in 1960 in the original cohort to 2488 Kcal/day in 1988) in this sample appeared, along with significant changes in the composition of the diet. Between 1960 and 1988 the consumption of bread had decreased by 70%, that of potatoes by 53%, of eggs by 48%, and of fruits by 31%; in contrast, fish consumption increased by 88%, that of meat by 160%, and that of cheese by 366%. Consumption of cereals, pulses, and sugar products had not changed significantly, whereas that of alcohol decreased by 33%. These changes brought about an increase in saturated fatty acid (S) intake of 27.5% and a simultaneous decrease of monounsaturated fatty acid (M) intake of 34% over 28 years. As a result of these changes, the ratio of polyunsaturated to saturated (P/S) fatty acids decreased from about 0.50 to 0.28 and the M/S ratio from 3.05 to 1.66 (Table 5) [5,10].

A recent meta-analysis [11] of six case-control studies carried out in the 1980s in Athens on a total of 228 men and 610 women 40–79 years old, all sedentary or hospitalized for fractures, presented the following pattern for urban subjects:

Table 4. Food consumption patterns in Cretan men, 1960 and 1988.

Food items	1960 (g/day) (n = 31)	1988[a] (g/day) (n = 182)	P
Bread	380	114.78 ± 79.78	<0.001
Cereals	30	29.09 ± 81.23	NS
Potatoes	190	88.35 ± 130.03	<0.001
Pulses	30	40.52 ± 108.16	NS
Vegetables	191	238.34 ± 196.31	<0.01
Fruits	464	322.31 ± 313.17	<0.001
Meat	35	91.20 ± 117.76	<0.001
Fish	18	34.04 ± 73.69	<0.01
Eggs	25	13.08 ± 44.45	<0.01
Cheese	13	60.58 ± 75.89	<0.001
Milk	235	57.84 ± 116.68	<0.001
Edible fats	95	49.96 ± 39.64	<0.001
Sugar products	20	20.59 ± 169.35	NS
Pastries	—	64.59 ± 169.35	—
Alcohol, 100%	15	10.15 ± 19.86	<0.01
Remainder of diet	107	161.61 ± 221.88	<0.001

[a] $x \pm$ SD. No standard deviations were reported for 1960; thus comparisons are one-sample t tests.
Data from [5,10].

Table 5. Dietary energy derived from fat in Cretan men, 1960 and 1988.

Item	1960 (n = 31) (ages 40–59 yr)	1988 (n = 181) (ages 40–60 yr)
Total calories (Kcal/d)	2685	2488
Total fat (g)	119.3	98.9
S fatty acids (g)	26.2	28.4
M fatty acids (g)	80.0	46.9
P fatty acids (g)	13.1	8.2
P/S ratio	0.50	0.28
M/S ratio	3.05	1.66
Total fat (% energy)	40	35.8
S fatty acids (% energy)	8	10.2
M fatty acids (% energy)	29	17.0
P fatty acids (% energy)	3	3.0
Cholesterol intake	125 mg/1000 Kcal/d	110 mg/1000 Kcal/d

S, saturated; M, monounsaturated; P, polyunsaturated.
Data from [5,10].

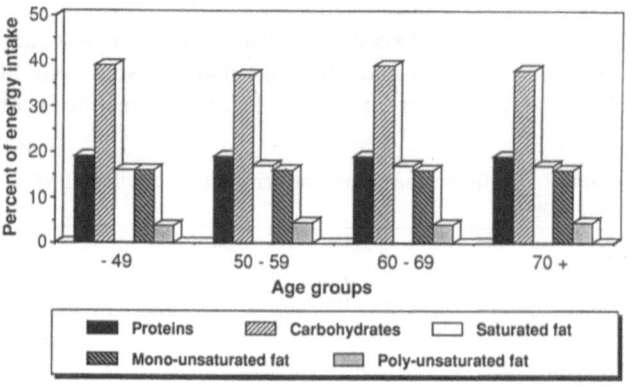

Fig. 10. Energy intake among urban men in Greece. (From [11], with permission)

(a) total energy intake (men, 1741 Kcal/day; women, 1409 Kcal/day) showed a mild declining trend with age, especially in women; (b) the percent of energy derived from proteins was about 19%, from carbohydrates about 37%, and from fats about 42% in men and 46% in women; (c) S fatty acids supplied 17% of energy in men and 19% in women, and the P/S/M ratio was about 1:4:4 (Fig. 10) [11].

The authors conclude that the contemporary Greek *urban* diet is still a high-fat diet. Thus, low-fat intake cannot be responsible for the apparently health-promoting consequences of this diet. They further point out that there may be an underestimation of olive oil intake and consequently of M fatty acid intake in all studies of the Greek diet, since olive oil, they note, "is regularly, liberally, and without special thought added in most Greek dishes." Nevertheless, these data provide evidence of the increasing amount of protein consumed, along with a definite increasing trend in saturated fat consumption, particularly in metropolitan areas of Greece, over the last 30 years.

Smoking

As a tobacco-producing country, Greece has one of the highest consumptions of tobacco products in the world. In 1965, Greece held the 15th position in cigarette consumption per capita (1950 cigarettes/persons per year): 17 years later (1982) it had climbed to second place (behind Cyprus and before Cuba), with 2927 cigarettes/person per year. A determined antismoking campaign in 1979–1981 by the late Minister of Health, S. Doxiades, attempting to arrest this trend, resulted in moderate success in 1980–1982. The change of government in 1981, however, and the stopping by the Ministry of Health of all campaigns for promotion of healthier lifestyles, apparently has restored the upward trend in tobacco consumption (Fig. 11) [4].

Among EC countries, Greece is first in the yearly consumption of cigarettes per person over age 15 years (Fig. 12) and second behind Denmark in the percentage of smokers in the adult population (43% vs 45%). Epidemiological studies indicate that the prevalence of smokers among high school graduates (17–18 years old) is 43% and among students of technological institutions this percentage reaches 60%, although very recent (unpublished) data indicate a tendency toward a reduction in the number of young smokers.

Regular smokers have an all-cause mortality rate approximately 50% higher than that of nonsmoking controls, and the excess deaths attributed to smoking can be calculated. In Europe, Greece occupies the second-highest position

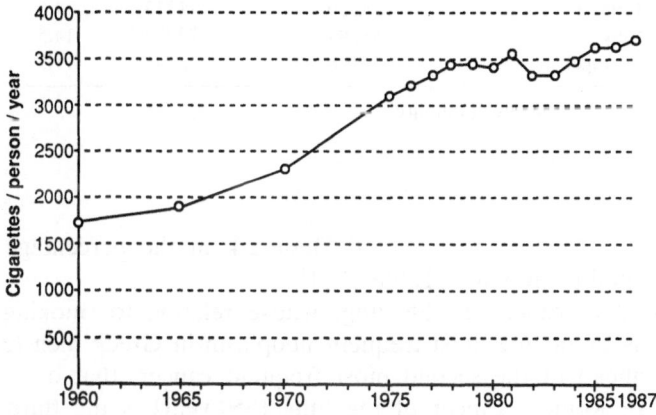

Fig. 11. Cigarette consumption in Greece per year per person older than 15 years. (From [4], with permission)

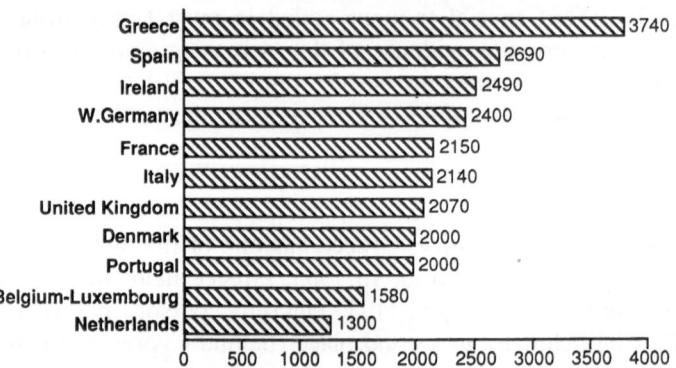

Fig. 12. Cigarette consumption in EC countries per year per person older than 15 years, 1987. (From [4], with permission)

Table 6. Yearly number of deaths attributed to smoking in subjects aged 25 years or more in EC countries (1986 or 1987).

Country	Number of deaths	Deaths attributed to smoking	
		Number	Percent
Denmark	56646	10423	18.4
Greece	88873	15731	17.7
Netherlands	122000	21594	17.7
France	530343	84855	16.0
Spain	287701	46032	16.0
West Germany	673835	103097	15.3
United Kingdom	629574	96325	15.3
Luxemburg	3953	605	15.3
Belgium	109199	16271	14.9
Ireland	32501	4713	14.5
Italy	532947	77277	14.5
Portugal	90783	10440	11.5

EC, European Community.
Data from [4].

(along with the Netherlands) behind Denmark in the percentage of excess deaths attributed to smoking (Table 6) [4].

With regard to cancer of the lung, whose relation to smoking is widely accepted, it is by far the most frequent neoplasm in Greek men (3400 cases/ year), well ahead of the second most frequent cancer, that of the stomach (780/year). In women, cancer of the lung (550/year) is the third most frequent cause, following breast and stomach, with 1190 and 580 cases per year, respectively.

Alcohol Consumption

The importance of alcohol as a risk factor for health is based on the relation between alcohol and a number of diseases and conditions which affect personal health, family, and social welfare. In conjunction with smoking, alcohol influences liver cirrhosis, certain neoplastic diseases, and traffic accidents. Information on alcohol "consumption" in various countries, however, is of limited value because the distinction between production and consumption is often impossible to make. Thus the data are only indicative.

Greece is a wine-producing country, but the traditional use of alcohol only by adult men during meals or social gatherings differs significantly from that of northern European countries. Within the European community, Greece occupies the last position in per capita alcohol consumption (8.7 l/year), about 59% that of Italy and 50% that of France. Curiously, it occupies also the last position in the proportion of abstainers (11%). The sources of alcohol are wine (54%), strong alcoholic beverages (30%), and beer (16%). During the period 1970–1981 the per capita alcohol consumption increased by 15%, but it has remained stable since, and it is estimated that there will be no major changes in the next few years [12].

Habitual Physical Activity

Very few studies on exact trends in physical activity of Greeks have been undertaken in the last 30 years, although it is apparent that physical activity among rural men has markedly decreased with the mechanization and automation of farming procedures.

In a 1991 resurvey of the surviving men of the original cohort of Crete (Kafatos et al., personal communication, 1994), 48 men aged 55–59 had significantly less frequent heavy physical activity compared with men aged 55–59 in 1960 (38.1% vs 64.2%) and more frequent sedentary or light physical activity (14.3% vs 5.4%; $P < 0.01$).

In the early 1960s, urban Cretans were reported to walk an average of 2–4 km/day [13]. In a 1982 study of 332 men farmers living in three villages near the Cretan villages originally studied, 86.3% reported having heavy physical activity [8]. In 1988, however, 70% of Cretan urban/suburban bank employees were sedentary, 20% walked 2–4 km/day, and only 10% practiced physical exercise daily [10]. These data are indicative of the diminished physical activity among the general Cretan population and probably apply to the larger urban/suburban population of Greece as a whole.

Risk Factors

Cholesterol

A number of studies have reported total cholesterol levels and fractions in several population groups throughout Greece since the 1960s. These studies

Table 7. Median values of total serum cholesterol (mg%) of middle-aged Greek men in five surveys 1960–1991.

Age	Crete 1960[a] (Men)	Crete 1982[a] (Men)	Crete 1988[b] (Men)	Crete 1991[c] (Men)	Athens 1979–81[d] (Men)	Athens 1979–81[d] (Women)
40–44	197.6	208.6	254.8	—	245.6	231.6
45–49	198.4	214.6		—	253.3	243.3
50–54	209.6	214.6	243.2	—	253.9	262.7
55–59	207.3	216.5		235.5	252.9	257.7
No. of subjects	652	239	163	48	729	953

[a] Data from [8].
[b] Data from [10].
[c] Kafatos et al., 1993, unpublished data.
[d] Data from [14].

generally agree that the levels found in 1960 have been exceeded. Because the methodology used was not the same, either in the fasting or nonfasting state of the subjects or in the chemical or enzymatic method employed, the data are not strictly comparable.

Within each study, however, age trends give important information about the groups examined. Table 7 [8,10,14] indicates the age trends of total serum cholesterol in five studies, four of which refer to rural or semirural populations of Crete between the 1960s and 1991 and one to a large study of Athenian men and women in 1979–1981. Peak levels are found in the age group 50–54, and the levels appear higher in more recent studies. Particularly elevated values are found in the Athenian men and women, having an average cholesterol level higher by 6.0 mg/dl at every age between 40 and 59 years than the values of American subjects of the same ages in the Pooling Project [15].

Systolic Blood Pressure (SBP) Levels

Table 8 presents median SBP levels in four studies between 1960 and 1991, the first three on the Cretan cohort and the fourth on a large Athenian sample in 1979–1981. Within each study an upward trend is apparent with increasing age. There is no trend toward higher values in more recent studies. Methodological rather than real differences may account for some puzzling findings (e.g., lower SBP in groups with higher body mass index [BMI]) [8].

In a 1987 study of 631 adults from two rural island communities, one of which experienced recently a marked socioeconomic tourist-related development, BMI and SBP levels, as well as serum cholesterol and smoking habits, were all higher in the community with the greater development [16].

Finally, in a 1991 resurvey of survivors of the original Cretan cohort, the mean SBP at ages 55–59, 70–79, and 80–89 years was 142.9, 157.7, and 165.3 mmHg, respectively (Kafatos et al., personal communication, 1994). The

Table 8. Median values of SBP (mmHg) in five studies on middle-aged Greek men and women 1960–91.

Age	Crete 1960[a] (Men)	Crete 1982[a] (Men)	Crete 1988[b] (Men)	Crete 1991[c] (Men)	Athens 1979–81[d] (Men)	Athens 1979–81[d] (Women)
40–44	131	125	128.6	—	123.8	119.1
45–49	132	120		—	127.8	127.7
50–54	135	125	131.8	—	133.9	133.7
55–59	138	130		142.9	137.0	138.3
No. of subjects	652	239	163	48	729	953

SBP, systemic blood pressure.
[a] Data from [8].
[b] Data from [10].
[c] Kafatos et al., 1993, unpublished data.
[d] Data from [14].

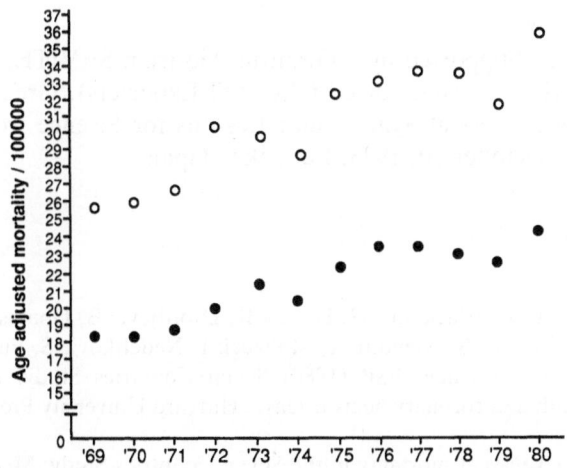

Fig. 13. Age-adjusted mortality from diabetes mellitus in Greek men (*closed circles*), and Greek women (*open circles*), 1969–1980. (From [6], with permission)

contribution of SBP changes over time to CHD mortality appears to be significant in the original Cretan and Corfu cohorts, in contrast to all other risk factors [17].

Body Mass Index

A sharp increase of BMI has appeared in all studies carried out in Greece subsequent to 1960. The frequency of severely overweight subjects (BMI ≥ 30 kg/m²) has increased about tenfold in Crete between 1960 and 1982 [8].

Most recent studies point to an average BMI in middle-aged men of $27.0\,kg/m^2$, which has remained relatively stable over the past 20 or more years [9]. The impact of this factor on CHD mortality is not significant, however, in recent analyses [17] (Keys et al., personal communication, 1994).

The common disease related to diet and obesity is diabetes mellitus (DM). Few data are available on the prevalence of DM in Greek population segments and the changes therein over the past 30 years. Among the few studies on prevalence of DM at the population level, a large-scale survey of 21359 home-dwelling inhabitants (10186 men, 11173 women) of an Athens suburb in 1974, repeated in 1990 on 12836 subjects (6252 men, 6584 women), indicated prevalence rates of 2.4% and 3.1% (age- and sex-standardized), respectively, of known DM. The increases were larger and the difference was more significant at ages progressively greater than 50 years [18].

Finally, Fig. 13 indicates the progressive increase in age-adjusted mortality per 100000 from DM in Greece by gender. These data support the epidemiological findings of increased prevalence of clinical DM [6].

Acknowledgments. Supported by a Grant-in-Aid from SEVITEL (Association of Greek Industries of Standardized Olive Oil Exporters), Greece. Presented in part at the International Symposium: Lessons for Science from the Seven Countries Study. October 30, 1993, Fukuoka, Japan.

References

1. Keys A, Aravanis C, Blackburn H, Buzina R, Djordjevic B, Dontas A, Fidanza F, Karvonen M, Kimura N, Menotti A, Mohacek I, Nedeljkovic S, Puddu V, Punsar S, Taylor H, van Buchem FSP (1980) Seven Countries Study. A multivariate analysis of death and coronary heart disease. Harvard University Press, Cambridge, Mass.
2. Keys A (1981) Ten-year mortality in the Seven Countries Study. Medical aspects of mortality statistics. Almqvist and Wiksell, Stockholm, pp 15–36
3. Menotti A, Keys A, Aravanis C, Blackburn H, Dontas A, Fidanza F, Karvonen MJ, Kromhout D, Nedeljkovic S, Nissinen A, Pekkanen J, Punsar S, Seccareccia F, Toshima H (1989) Seven Countries Study. First 20-year mortality data in 12 cohorts of six countries. Ann Med 21:175–179
4. Kalapothaki V, Kalantidi A, Katsouyanni K, Trichopoulou A, Kyriopoulos J, Kremastinou J, Hadjiconstantinou V, Trichopoulos D (1992) The health of the Greek population (in Greek). Materia Med Greca 20:91–164
5. Keys A, Aravanis C, Sdrin H (1966) Diets of middle-aged men in two rural areas of Greece. Voeding 27:575–586
6. Trichopoulou A, Efstathiadis P (1989) Changes of nutrition patterns and health indicators at the population level in Greece. Am J Clin Nutr 49:1042–1047
7. Kafatos AG, Christakis G, Hsià SL, Cassady J, Panagiotakopoulos G (1980) Serum lipid levels in 1010 Greek children, age 10–14 years (in Greek). Iatriki 38:283–290

8. Aravanis C, Mensink RP, Corcondilas A, Ioannidis P, Feskens EJM, Katan MB (1988) Risk factors for coronary heart disease in middle-aged men in Crete in 1982. Int J Epidemiol 17:779–783
9. Kromhout D, Keys A, Aravanis C, Buzina R, Fidanza F, Giampaoli S, Jansen A, Menotti A, Nedeljkovic S, Pekkarinen M, Simic BS, Toshima H (1989) Food consumption patterns in the 1960s in seven countries. Am J Clin Nutr 49:889–894
10. Kafatos A, Kouroumalis I, Vlachonikolis I, Theodorou C, Labadarios D (1991) Coronary heart disease risk factor status of the Cretan urban population in the 1980s. Am J Clin Nutr 54:591–598
11. Trichopoulou A, Toupadaki N, Tzonou A, Katsouyanni K, Manousos O, Kada E, Trichopoulos D (1993) The macronutrient composition of the Greek diet: estimates derived from six case-control studies. Eur J Clin Nutr 47:549–558
12. Trichopoulos D (1989) New patterns of alcohol consumption and health effects. A report to the EEC: Directorate General: Employment, Social Affairs and Education
13. Christakis G, Severinghaus EL, Maldonado Z, Kafatos FC, Hashim SA (1965) Crete: a study in the metabolic epidemiology of coronary heart disease. Am J Cardiol 15:320–332
14. Moulopoulos SD, Adamopoulos PN, Diamantopoulos EI, Nanas SN, Anthopoulos LN, Iliadi-Alexandrou M (1987) Coronary heart disease risk factors in a random sample of Athenian adults; the Athens Study. Am J Epidemiol 126:882–892
15. Pooling Project Research Group (1978) Relationship of blood pressure serum cholesterol, smoking habit, relative weight, and ECG abnormalities to incidence of major coronary events: final report of the Pooling Project. American Heart Association, Monograph no. 60
16. Adamopoulos PN, Boutsicakis J, Kodoyanis S, Papamichael C, Gatos A, Makrilakis K, Argyros D, Adamopoulos E, Argyros G, Kostis F, Economou D, Iliadou-Alexandrou M (1990) Blood pressure and other risk factors of cardiovascular disease in two communities with different socio-economic statuses: the Athens Study. J Human Hyperten 4:344–349
17. Dontas AS, Menotti A, Aravanis C, Corcondilas A, Lekos D, Seccareccia F (1993) Long-term prediction of coronary heart disease mortality in two rural Greek populations. Eur Heart J 14:1153–1157
18. Katsilambros N, Aliferis K, Darviri CH, Tsapogas P, Alexiou Z, Tritos N, Arvanitis M (1993) Evidence for an increase in the prevalence of known diabetes in a sample of an urban population in Greece. Diabet Med 10:87–90

Recent Trends in Cardiovascular Disease and Risk Factors in the Seven Countries: Italy

ALESSANDRO MENOTTI and SIMONA GIAMPAOLI[1]

Summary. Between 1969 and 1990, Italy experienced a marked decline in cardiovascular disease death rates. In particular, rates from coronary heart disease decreased by 40% in men and 51% in women; rates from cerebro-vascular disease decreased by 43% in men and 41% in women; and rates from cardiovascular diseases overall decreased by 42% in men and 48% in women. Large-scale population surveys on the main cardiovascular risk factors per-formed on middle-aged people (aged 30–59 years) in 1978–1979, 1983–1984, and 1985–1987 showed a significant decline in mean levels of blood pressure (in both sexes), in body mass index (in women), and in cigarette smoking (in men), while serum cholesterol remained substantially unchanged. With the use of risk functions generated from Italian population studies, it was shown that about two-thirds of the decline in cardiovascular mortality was mathematically "explained" by the observed risk factor changes. It is assumed that part of the mortality decline is due to improved medical and surgical treatment and to rehabilitation of cardiovascular diseases.

Key words. Cardiovascular diseases—Risk factor changes—Mortality trends—Italy

Introduction

The recent changes observed in death rates from cardiovascular, mainly cor-onary, disease in many countries started about 25 years ago in the United States, soon followed by declines in other industrialized countries [1–4]. On the other hand, until recently, death rates in the countries of Eastern Europe, and in many other nonindustrialized countries, continued to rise. Interna-tional conferences held in Bethesda, Maryland in 1978 [1] and 1988 [5] tried to establish whether such changes were true and whether they could be explained.

Among the western industrialized countries, Italy showed upward trends until the late 1970s [6], and only then, about 10 years later than in the United

States and elsewhere, did a marked decline in deaths become evident [7,8]. A review of the present status of the issue is given here.

Materials and Methods

In Italy official mortality data are collected by the Italian National Institute of Statistics, while estimates of the resident population in the years between the decennial censuses, and computation of official death rates, are made by the Italian National Institute of Health, whose data bank has been consulted for the purpose. Official numerators, denominators, and rates become available in Italy with a delay of about 3 years after a given year of observation. Detailed information is now available from 1969 to 1990. For the purpose of this analysis, we considered the following groupings of causes of death, as identified by the corresponding codes of the World Health Organization, *International Classification of Diseases*, Ninth Revision [9], (for the years preceding the use of the Ninth Revision, the Eighth Revision [10] was employed after adjustments made to provide full comparability with the Ninth):

Ischemic heart diseases: codes 410–414 (called coronary heart disease)
Cerebrovascular disease: codes 430–438 (called strokes)
All cardiovascular diseases: codes 390–459 (called cardiovascular diseases)
All-cause mortality: codes 001–999, taken as reference for some analyses

Death rates for each of these causes were computed for each year from 1969 to 1990, separately for men and women and for quinquennia of age 0–4, 6–9, 10–14, and so on until age 95–99. The quinquennial death rates were then compacted into age-adjusted death rates for the following age ranges: 0–99, 30–59, 40–69, 65–99. The reason for those ranges will become clear in the chapter on results. The age adjustment was made by direct standardization, taking as reference the age distribution of the Italian population from the census of 1981 in the proper age ranges, whose information is incorporated in the same data bank. The death rates were expressed per 100 000 population.

The time trends in cardiovascular mortality have been correlated against the time changes in cardiovascular risk factors derived from three major studies on population samples conducted in Italy between the late 1970s and the late 1980s. The first study (RF2) was conducted in 1978–1979 among nine samples of men and women located in nine different health districts (out of over 600 in Italy) in eight different regions [11,12]. It included people aged 20–59, but for the purpose of this analysis only people aged 30–59 were considered. The nine areas included locations in northern, central, southern, and insular Italy, characterized by both urban and rural environments. They did not necessarily represent the whole country, but were representative of many similar localities.

The second study (OB43) was conducted in 1983-1984 in the same nine health districts where independent samples were drawn, and the same age selection was made for the purpose of this analysis [13,14].

The third study (MICOL), conducted in 1985-1987, covered 18 population samples of men and women aged 30-69 from 18 different health districts in ten different regions [8,15]. The primary interest was the epidemiology of gallstones, but some major cardiovascular risk factors were also measured. For the purpose of this analysis, only people aged 30-59 were considered. Geographically speaking, the 18 areas in the MICOL study did not correspond exactly to the 9 investigated in the two previous studies. However, they represented more regions (i.e., 10), some of which coincided with those of the other two studies and a large variety of Italian socioeconomic groups were included.

Measurements were made of height, weight, total serum cholesterol, and systolic (SBP) and diastolic blood pressure (DBP), and information was taken on cigarette consumption and on the use of antihypertensive drugs, following the same rules and quality control procedures described in detail elsewhere [9,11-15]. Briefly, height and weight were measured without shoes and in light underwear following the technique described by the WHO *Manual on Cardiovascular Survey Methods* [16] (from now on called the WHO *Manual*). Height and weight were then used to compute body mass index (kg/m^2).

Blood pressure was measured in the right arm, in a sitting position after 4 min rest, by trained and tested observers following the procedure described by the WHO *Manual* [16]. Measurements were taken to the nearest 2 mmHg using standard mercury sphygmomanometers. Diastolic pressure corresponded to the fifth phase of the Korotkoff sounds, and for the analysis the average of two consecutive measurements was used. Training and testing of the observers was performed using the procedure and the cassettes of the London School of Hygiene.

Serum cholesterol was measured on fresh sera drawn from subjects fasting 12 h. Different enzymatic automated techniques were employed in the different centers, but all of them were under the quality control of a central laboratory in Italy and (directly or indirectly) of the WHO Lipid Reference Center of Prague.

Information on smoking was obtained through a questionnaire derived from that proposed by the WHO *Manual* [16].

Two questions were asked on the current use of antihypertensive drugs, with a check on their commercial name. This information is comparable only between studies RF2 and OB43.

The three studies were coordinated by the Istituto Superiore di Sanita, Rome (Italian National Institute of Health). Detailed data on the distribution and mean levels of these selected risk factors were reported elsewhere [8, 11-15]. The risk-factor levels were treated as age-standardized means (taking as reference the age distribution of the appropriate age range from the 1981 Italian census) or as age-standardized proportions (for cigarette smokers).

The coefficients of three proportional hazards models generated from another Italian population sample were used to compute a combined estimate of the risk of death from coronary heart disease, from cerebrovascular disease, and from all cardiovascular diseases. The factors employed in the prediction were age, mean blood pressure (diastolic plus one third of the difference between systolic and diastolic blood pressure), serum cholesterol, the number of cigarettes smoked per day, and body mass index. The models were obtained from the only Italian long-term population study to produce reliable risk functions for the prediction of mortality [17]. The population comprised 1551 men originally aged 40–59, and then followed up for 25 years. The coefficients for coronary heart disease were: age 0.0171; cholesterol 0.0072; mean blood pressure 0.0315; cigarettes 0.0186; body mass index −0.0052. The coefficients for cerebrovascular diseases were: age 0.1222; cholesterol 0.0056; mean blood pressure 0.0373; cigarettes 0.0053; body mass index −0.0704. The coefficients for all cardiovascular diseases were: age 0.1083; cholesterol 0.0065; mean blood pressure 0.0317; cigarettes 0.0156; body mass index −0.0270. The values of t_0 were chosen for a period of five years and were 0.9929, 0.9976, and 0.9861 for coronary heart disease, strokes, and all cardiovascular diseases, respectively.

With the composite estimate of risk for selected periods of time and selected age ranges, an attempt was made to estimate the proportion of the decline explained hypothetically by the risk-factor changes.

Results

Tables 1–4 summarize the death rate changes that occurred in Italy between 1969 and 1990. For coronary heart disease, the peak year for the majority of the age-sex groups was sometime in the 1970s. Dramatic changes occurred afterward, with a decline greater than 30% in men and greater than 40% and

Table 1. Trends in mortality from coronary heart disease[a] in Italy between 1969 and 1990.

Sex	Age	Rates (Age-adjusted, per 100 000)				Change (%)	
		1969	1990	Peak	Year of peak	1969–1990	Peak–1990
M	0–99	170	115	191	1978	−32	−40
M	30–59	86	53	98	1978	−38	−46
M	40–69	213	146	236	1978	−31	−38
M	65–99	1100	750	1240	1978	−32	−39
F	0–99	145	77	156	1973	−47	−51
F	30–59	20	10	20	1969	−50	−50
F	40–69	75	39	75	1969	−48	−48
F	65–99	870	460	960	1973	−47	−52

[a] World Health Organization *International Classification of Diseases* codes 410–414.

up to 50% in women. The benefit was substantial also in the elderly of both sexes.

It is known that some decline in stroke deaths occurred before 1969, but after that date the decline was continuous. Again, the advantage was larger among women (37%–42%) than among men (28%–34%). Also, in this case a large decrease in stroke mortality was observed among the elderly.

In the wider group of cardiovascular diseases, the trend was also downward from 1969, involving women (46%–63%) more than men (41%–46%). It benefited also the elderly.

As reference, data on all-cause mortality are given in Table 4. It appears that the marked decrease in all-cause death rates is largely explained by the decline in cardiovascular mortality, which was, and remains, the first cause of death in Italy. At the same time, it is known that the second major cause of death (cancer) did not show any decrease, but rather increased in the same period of time, while declining mortality rates occurred in a number of less frequent causes of death.

Table 2. Trends in mortality from strokes[a] in Italy between 1969 and 1990.

Sex	Age	Rates (Age-adjusted, per 100 000)				Change (%)	
		1969	1990	Peak	Year of peak	1969–1990	Peak–1990
M	0–99	145	82	145	1969	−43	−43
M	30–59	35	18	35	1969	−49	−49
M	40–69	124	59	124	1969	−52	−52
M	65–99	1100	63	1110	1969	−43	−43
F	0–99	171	100	171	1969	−41	−41
F	30–59	26	11	26	1969	−58	−58
F	40–69	93	36	93	1969	−61	−61
F	65–99	1020	610	1020	1969	−40	−40

[a] World Health Organization *International Classification of Diseases* codes 430–438.

Table 3. Trends in mortality from cardiovascular diseases[a] in Italy between 1969 and 1990.

Sex	Age	Rates (Age-adjusted, per 100 000)				Change (%)	
		1969	1990	Peak	Year of peak	1969–1990	Peak–1990
M	0–99	511	297	511	1969	−42	−42
M	30–59	179	97	179	1969	−46	−46
M	40–69	506	280	506	1969	−45	−45
M	65–99	3640	2140	3640	1969	−41	−41
F	0–99	570	298	570	1969	−48	−48
F	30–59	95	35	95	1969	−63	−63
F	40–69	303	118	303	1969	−61	−61
F	65–99	3380	1820	3380	1969	−46	−46

[a] World Health Organization *International Classification of Diseases* codes 390–459.

Table 4. Trends in mortality from all causes of death[a] in Italy between 1969 and 1990.

| Sex | Age | Rates (Age-adjusted, per 100000) | | | | Change (%) | |
		1969	1990	Peak	Year of peak	1969–1990	Peak–1990
M	0–99	1185	815	1185	1969	−31	−31
M	30–59	585	384	585	1969	−34	−34
M	40–69	1375	925	1375	1969	−33	−33
M	65–99	7060	505	7060	1969	−28	−28
F	0–99	1079	658	1079	1969	−39	−39
F	30–59	321	187	321	1969	−42	−42
F	40–69	759	446	759	1969	−41	−41
F	65–99	5660	3560	5660	1969	−37	−37

[a] World Health Organization *International Classification of Diseases* codes 001–999.

Table 5. Mean changes in some cardiovascular risk factors, expressed in original units, in three national surveys of men and women aged 30–59.

| | Entry level 1978–1979 | | Change | | | | | |
| | | | 1978–1979 to 1983–1984 | | 1983–1984 to 1985–1987 | | 1978–1979 to 1985–1987 | |
	M	F	M	F	M	F	M	F
Serum cholesterol (mg/dl)	220.4 ±47.9	213.8 ±44.0	+1.2	−1.1	−0.8	0	+0.4	−1.1
Systolic blood pressure (mmHg)	135.5 ±18.8	136.0 ±20.5	−1.2	−4.9	−2.1	−1.6	−3.3	−6.5
Diastolic blood pressure (mmHg)	87.1 ±11.5	85.8 ±11.5	−1.8	−3.3	−0.7	−0.3	−2.5	−3.6
Prevalence of smokers (%)	54.2 ±1.0	20.1 ±0.7	−5.0	+2.9	−5.5	+0.9	−10.5	+3.8
Cigarettes (n/day)	10.2 ±12.2	2.2 ±5.4	−0.7	+0.4	−1.3	+0.3	−2.0	+0.7
Body mass index (kg/m²)	25.9 ±3.5	26.3 ±4.8	+0.1	−0.9	+0.3	+0.3	+0.4	−0.6

An attempt to explain at least part of the decreasing death rates from cardiovascular diseases was made by exploiting the epidemiological material described in the section on materials and methods.

Table 5 summarizes the changes in mean levels of some cardiovascular risk factors observed in the three major national surveys conducted in 1978–1979, 1983–1984, and 1985–1987. They refer to both men and women aged 30–59. Small but distinct decreases occurred in mean systolic and diastolic blood pressure in both men and women, but were always more pronounced in women. Smoking habits, expressed by the prevalence of smokers and by the mean daily consumption of cigarettes in all people (smokers and nonsmokers), declined in men, while rising slightly in women. The prevalence of smokers among men declined from 54.2% to 43.7% in a 9-year period.

Body mass index was relatively stable or rose slightly in men while clearly decreasing among women. The absolute weight in women did not much change in the three surveys, but women were taller as new generations entered the samples.

Finally, no changes were seen in the mean levels of serum cholesterol, although the balance was reached by slight falls in some northern regions against rises in the southern ones.

The levels of cardiovascular risk-factors were entered into comprehensive estimates of risk, separately for coronary heart disease, strokes, and cardiovascular diseases, using the risk functions mentioned in the section on materials and methods. The changes of estimated risk were correlated against the change in national mortality rates. Since only three time points were available for risk-factors, the attempt to explain the mortality changes by risk-factor changes could be made only in relation to limited time periods.

Several options could be adopted. Finally, the following hypotheses were put forward:

1. It was hypothesized that the risk-factor changes between 1978–1979 and 1983–1984 affected the mortality rates of the period between 1983–1984 and 1985–1987.
2. It was hypothesized that the risk-factor changes between 1978–1979 and 1985–1987 affected the mortality rates of the period between 1985–1987 and 1990.

In both cases, the observed changes in risk-factors by generation were computed for people aged 30–59, with such changes projected on mortality of people aged both 30–59 and 40–69, in order to allow the time-lag effect of risk-factor changes to "act" on mortality. The death rates were used as averages when more than one calendar year was involved.

In Tables 6–8 the expected changes (estimated from risk-factor changes) are compared with the observed changes and the proportion of the changes "explained" is computed as expected/observed, times 100. For coronary heart disease, the "explained" decline varies in men from 45.7% to 71.9%, higher when the observed changes are those projected on the age range 40–69. Moreover, the risk-factor changes better explain the mortality changes when a longer period of risk-factor changes is considered (1978–1979 to 1985–1987 instead of 1978–1979 to 1983–1984). Roughly the same general considerations are true for women, but the overall proportions of mortality decline "explained" is higher (86.9%–98.9%).

For strokes, the "explained" differential mortality is altogether smaller than for coronary heart disease. The "explained" decline is not much different between men and women and ranges from 43.3% to 67.8%. With one exception, the better explanation is linked to longer exposure to risk-factor changes in the age range 40–69.

Table 6. Estimated coronary mortality risk reduction (based on risk-factor changes) and observed coronary mortality decline in defined periods for both sexes and two age ranges.

| Risk-factor changes[a] | | | | | | | Mortality changes | | |
Sex	From	To	Sex	Age	From	To	Expected (%)	Observed (%)	Explained (%)
M	1978–79	1983–84	M	30–59	1983–84	1985–87	−5.3	−11.6	45.7
M	1978–79	1985–87	M	30–59	1985–87	1990	−11.5	−20.1	57.2
M	1978–79	1983–84	M	40–69	1983–84	1985–87	−5.3	−8.4	63.1
M	1978–79	1985–87	M	40–69	1985–87	1990	−11.5	−16.1	71.9
F	1978–79	1983–84	F	30–59	1983–84	1985–87	−11.0	−10.0	90.9
F	1978–79	1985–87	F	30–59	1985–87	1990	−12.6	−14.5	86.9
F	1978–79	1983–84	F	40–69	1983–84	1985–87	−11.0	−11.5	95.6
F	1978–79	1985–87	F	49–69	1985–87	1990	−12.6	−12.8	98.4

[a] All risk-factor changes computed on age range 30–59.

Table 7. Estimated stroke mortality risk reduction (based on risk-factor changes) and observed stroke mortality decline in defined periods for both sexes and two age ranges.

| Risk-factor changes | | | | | | | Mortality changes | | |
Sex	From	To	Sex	Age	From	To	Expected (%)	Observed (%)	Explained (%)
M	1978–79	1983–84	M	30–59	1983–84	1985–87	−6.1	−13.2	46.2
M	1978–79	1985–87	M	30–59	1985–87	1990	−12.9	−25.9	49.8
M	1978–79	1983–84	M	40–69	1983–84	1985–87	−6.1	−14.1	43.3
M	1978–79	1985–87	M	40–69	1985–87	1990	−12.9	−21.5	60.0
F	1978–79	1983–84	F	30–59	1983–84	1985–87	−8.0	−11.8	67.8
F	1978–79	1985–87	F	30–59	1985–87	1990	−12.1	−26.7	45.3
F	1978–79	1983–84	F	40–69	1983–84	1985–87	−8.0	−17.6	45.4
F	1978–79	1985–87	F	49–69	1985–87	1990	−12.1	−20.5	59.0

[a] All risk-factor changes computed on age range 30–59.

Table 8. Estimated cardiovascular mortality risk reduction (based on risk-factor changes) and observed CHD mortality decline in defined periods for both sexes and two age ranges.

| Risk-factor changes | | | | | | | Mortality changes | | |
Sex	From	To	Sex	Age	From	To	Expected (%)	Observed (%)	Explained (%)
M	1978–79	1983–84	M	30–59	1983–84	1985–87	−5.4	−13.4	40.3
M	1978–79	1985–87	M	30–59	1985–87	1990	−11.8	−20.3	58.1
M	1978–79	1983–84	M	40–69	1983–84	1985–87	−5.4	−11.9	45.4
M	1978–79	1985–87	M	40–69	1985–87	1990	−11.8	−17.9	65.9
F	1978–79	1983–84	F	30–59	1983–84	1985–87	−13.2	−15.1	87.4
F	1978–79	1985–87	F	30–59	1985–87	1990	−15.4	−19.9	77.4
F	1978–79	1983–84	F	40–69	1983–84	1985–87	−13.2	−14.1	90.6
F	1978–79	1985–87	F	40–69	1985–87	1990	−15.4	−19.9	77.4

[a] All risk-factor changes computed on age range 30–59.

The picture for cardiovascular diseases is more like that for coronary heart disease than that for strokes. The proportions explained ranges from 40.3% to 65.9% for men and 77.4% to 90.6% for women. In men, again, a longer exposure to risk-factor changes and use of the age range 40–69 for observed mortality better "explains" the mortality changes. In women this is not true, but the proportion of decline "explained" is systematically greater.

Discussion

This analysis shows that death rates from cardiovascular diseases in Italy have greatly declined during a 10- to 12-year period. Such changes have been of the same order of magnitude as those recorded in the United States and elsewhere, where they started a decade in advance [5].

Unfortunately, in Italy there are uncertainties in the coding of causes of death, particularly in the area of cardiovascular diseases. Coronary heart disease and stroke cover about 65% of all cardiovascular deaths, the remaining 35% being mainly made up by a number of nonspecific diagnoses such as heart failure, atherosclerosis, hypertension, "collapse," etc., which may hide more specific conditions. These nonspecific diagnoses are more common among the elderly than younger age groups, among women than among men, and in the southern regions than in other regions of the country. The contribution of specific well-defined heart or circulatory diseases (such as cardiomyopathy, bacterial endocarditis, pulmonary heart disease, aneurysm, etc.) to this hetero-geneous group is marginal. As a consequence, the analysis was expanded to the whole of cardiovascular diseases to avoid possible bias due to uncertainties in death coding. The overall trends are similar for coronary heart diseases, stroke, and cardiovascular diseases.

The risk-factor changes between 1978–1979 and 1985–1987, derived from the three population studies employed here, is the most extensive information on the subject available in the country and therefore must be relied upon. The population samples involved, however, do not necessarily represent the whole country because they do not derive from national statistical samples.

The decline in mean levels of blood pressure partly reflects the documented increase in treatment and control of hypertension. In fact, the comparison of the 1978–1979 survey with the 1983–1984 survey showed a marked increase in the proportion of treated hypertensives [8]. However, this is not the only cause of the phenomenon, since in the more recent surveys a lower mean blood pressure was found also among the younger strata of the adult population, where the impact of hypertension treatment is negligible [8,13,14]. The reduc-tion in prevalence of smokers and mean cigarette consumption among men is somehow unexpected (although well-documented from other sources [18]) since major antismoking campaigns were never organized in Italy. The rising prevalence of smokers among women apparently reflects the consequence of the "liberation" of women. This will hopefully be attenuated in the next years.

The decreasing body mass index among females may be the consequence of the "cosmetic motivations" that have spread in the last two decades.

Finally, the overall stability of serum cholesterol levels, apart from the regional differences, is apparently in contrast to the increasing fat and calorie consumption recorded during the last decades [19]. A large amount of food waste has been documented, however, in ad hoc observations (A. Turchetto, personal communication, 1993).

The technique for "explaining" changes in mortality is approximate, through risk functions derived from populations examined first in the 1960s. On the other hand, more recent and more reliable risk functions are not yet available for Italy. Another problem is the use of risk functions from men for the estimate of cardiovascular risk in women, but no study in Italy was able to produce reliable risk functions for women. This means that the same risk-factor/mortality relationships were assumed valid for men and women.

Overall, the proportion of the decline in cardiovascular mortality explained by a few basic risk-factor changes is relatively high, ranging, according to the different estimates, from 40% to 70% for men and 40% to 90+% for women. The larger "explanation" for women's mortality may be biased by the use of non-sex-specific risk functions. As a consequence, caution should be taken in interpreting these data on women.

Altogether, when considering the time lag, the temporal sequence, and the age shift, the proportion of changes in mortality explained by risk-factor changes is statistically sound and biologically congruent. Other attempts, made without allowing a proper time lag (not reported here), show a smaller "explained" decline.

The overall modeling of risk-factor trends versus mortality trends could be improved if larger data bases were available on risk-factor changes. Large-scale surveys on risk factors at the national level were not performed after 1987, but scattered local studies in the early 1990s offered information. Within Area Brianza of the Monica Project (in northern Italy) [20], a decline in mean cholesterol levels was shown in the late 1980s. In two studies conducted in the Emilia (again northern Italy) [21], serum cholesterol and blood pressure showed clear-cut lower levels compared to surveys conducted in the same areas some years beforehand. The start of a decline in cholesterol levels recorded in northern Italy is consistent with several other facts: the highest levels of serum cholesterol were reached in northern Italy in the 1970s; that area exhibited the highest death rates from coronary (and cardiovascular) diseases; the mortality decline in northern Italy started before that in other areas of the country, in the same area where the first cholesterol falls were observed, whereas until the mid-1980s cholesterol levels in the southern part of the country were still increasing.

In a study conducted in Rome and Florence (central Italy) in the early 1990s on samples of men aged 40–59, the mean levels of blood pressure, of cigarette consumption and the prevalence of smokers were even lower than those

Table 9. Heart disease facilities and activities in Italy (population 57 million).

	Number	Year	Notes
Hospital divisions and services of cardiology	513	1986	1st division in 1956
Hospital beds for cardiac patients	6966	1986	—
Coronary care units (CCU)	249	1986	1st CCU in 1966
Beds in CCU	1469	1986	—
Cardiac surgery units	54	1990	—
Coronary bypass surgery	10, 340	1990	About 1/4 compared with United States
Cardiac rehabilitation units	64	1990	1st CRU in 1968

Data from [22, 23].

recorded in the national survey of 1985–1987, in an altogether younger age group, 30–59 (F. Seccareccia, personal communication, 1993).

The "explained decline" found in this analysis is consistent with similar conclusions offered by other studies where from one-half to two-thirds of the mortality decline phenomenon could be attributed to risk-factor trends.

Proper models for evaluation of the role of treatment versus prevention are not available. Usually the role of treatment has been estimated by the difference in the total decline minus the proportion attributable to risk factors [1,5]. The same applies to Italy, and only anecdotal information can be provided. In a total population now close to 57 million, the number of coronary care units increased from none in the mid-1960s to about 250 now. In recent years, coronary bypass surgery has been performed on over 10 000 subjects per year; the use of beta-blockers, calcium antagonists, angiotensin-converting enzyme (ACE) inhibitors, and thrombolysis became widespread all over the country; centers for cardiac rehabilitation increased from none in the 1960s to more than 60 in 1990 [22,23] (Table 10).

All this indicates that a contribution to the mortality decline of treatment of established coronary heart disease is clear, but quantification cannot be modelled.

Many more difficulties are encountered when trying to describe real improvements in the treatment of stroke, where information and data are scanty.

On the other hand, all the changes described refer only to mortality, since data on incidence are not available. Modelled projections made on the basis of scattered Italian incidence data suggest a reduction in the occurrence of new cases (A. Verdecchia, personal communication, 1993), whereas the Monica Project, in which Italy participates [24], has produced, so far, no clear-cut evidence of changing incidence.

Presently the picture seems favorable, although much more can be done for improving cardiovascular health in this country. The legacy and tradition of the Mediterranean diet and lifestyle were apparently never completely lost, and now this pattern undergoes a revival. All this probably contributed to the increasing life expectancy of the Italian population, now approaching that of countries at the highest rank all over the world.

Acknowledgments. Research partly developed within the Italian National Research Council (CNR) targeted project "Prevention and Control of Disease Factors" (FATMA), subproject "Community Medicine", CNR Contract 93.00773.PF41.

References

1. U.S. Department of Health, Education and Welfare (1979) Proceedings of the Conference on the Decline in Coronary Heart Disease Mortality. U.S. Department of Health, Education and Welfare, Public Health Service, National Institutes of Health, Publ No. 70-1610
2. Pisa Z, Uemura K (1982) Trends of mortality from ischaemic disease and other cardiovascular disease in 27 countries 1968–1977. WHO Stat Q 35:11–47
3. Uemura K, Pisa Z (1985) Recent trends in cardiovascular mortality in 27 industrialized countries. WHO Stat Q 38:142–162
4. Uemura K, Pisa Z (1988) Trends in cardiovascular disease mortality in industrialized countries since 1950. WHO Stat Q 41:155–178
5. Higgins MW, Luepker RV (eds) (1989) Trends and determinants of coronary heart disease mortality. International comparisons. Int J Epidemiol 18[Suppl I]:S1–S232
6. Menotti A, Capocaccia R, Farchi G, Pasquali M (1985) Recent trends in coronary heart disease and other cardiovascular disease in Italy. Cardiology 72:88–96
7. Menotti A (1989) Trends in CHD in Italy. Int J Epidemiol 18[Suppl I]:S125–S128
8. Menotti A, Scanga M, and the Responsible Investigators of the RF2, OB43, and the MICOL Research Groups (1992) Recent trends in selected coronary risk factors in Italy. Int J Epidemiol 21:883–892
9. World Health Organization (1977) International classification of diseases, 9th rev. World Health Organization, Geneva
10. World Health Organization (1965) International classification of diseases, 8th rev. World Health Organization, Geneva
11. Gruppo di Ricerca ATS-RF2 (1980) I fattori di rischio dell'arteriosclerosi in Italia. La fase A del progetto finalizzato del CNR Medicina Preventiva-Aterosclerosi-RF2. G It Cardiol 10[Suppl III]:1–184
12. Research Group ATS-RF2 of the Italian National Research Council (1981) Distribution of some risk factors for atherosclerosis in nine Italian population samples. Am J Epidemiol 113:338–346
13. Gruppo di Ricerca ATS-OB43 (1987) I fattori di rischio cardiovascolare in Italia. Aggiornamento agli anni '80 dello studio delle nove comunità. Riv Card Prev Riab 5:75–137
14. Research Group ATS-RF2-OB43 of the Italian National Research Council (1987) Time trends of some cardiovascular risk factors in Italy. Am J Epidemiol 126:95–103
15. The MICOL Group (1991) Prevalence of gall-bladder disease in 18 Italian population samples. First results from the MICOL Study. In: Capocaccia L, et al. (eds)

Recent advances in the epidemiology and prevention of gall-bladder disease. Kluwer Academic Publishers, Dordrecht, Netherlands, pp 37–44

16. Rose GA, Blackburn H (1968) Cardiovascular survey methods. World Health Organization, Geneva
17. Menotti A, Mariotti S, Seccareccia F, Giampaoli S (1988) The 25-year estimated probability of death from some specific causes as a function of twelve risk factors in middle-aged men. Eur J Epidemiol 4:60–67
18. Menotti A, Seccareccia F (1990) Fumatori e non: ultimi dati sull'accorciamento della vita. In: Atti VII Simposio del Centro per la lotta contro l'Infarto. Ciba-Geigy, Florence, pp 251–256
19. Istituto Nazionale della Nutrizione (1992) Alimentazione e Nutrizione in Italia: aspetti, problemi, proposte. International FAO-WHO Conference on Nutrition, National Institute of Nutrition, Rome, pp 1–94
20. Cesana G, Ferrario M, Sega R, Bravi C, Gussoni MT, De Vito G, Valagussa F (1992) Declino della mortalita cardiovascolare e coronarica in Lombardia, 1969–1987. Valutazione della affidabilità delle stime e possibili ipotesi esplicative. G Ital Cardiol 22:293–305
21. D'Addato S, Barozzi G, Benassi B and 25 collaborators (1992) Indagine sui fattori di rischio cardiovascolare in un campione di popolazione di Bologna. Giorn Arterioscle 17:155–162
22. De Vita C, Lotto A, Mazzari FM, Vecchio C (1989) La prevenzione secondaria e la riabilitazione cardilogica. G Ital Cardiol 19(9):119–125
23. Boncompagni F, Pesciatini F, Cafiero M, Ignone GF, Mazzalini M, Sala L, Scardi S (1992) La riabilitazione del cardiopatico operato in Italia: realtà attuale e prospettive future. G Riabil (Rome) 8:311–314

Recent Trends in Cardiovascular Disease and Risk Factors in the Seven Countries: The Netherlands

W.M. Monique Verschuren, Henriette A. Smit, Edith M. van Leer, Jacob C. Seidell, and Daan Kromhout[1]

Summary. This chapter describes trends in total cholesterol, blood pressure, cigarette smoking, and body mass index in the Netherlands. Data from three screening projects are available, carried out consecutively in the periods 1974–1980 (men and women aged 37–43 years), 1981–1986 (men aged 33–37 years), and 1987–1991 (men and women aged 20–59 years). For smoking, data are available since 1958. For total cholesterol no substantial changes have taken place in the general population. The prevalence of hypertension has remained more or less stable, while treatment of hypertension has decreased since 1987. A decrease in cigarette smoking in men was strongest in the 1970s, slowed down considerably in the 1980s, and has almost come to a standstill in the 1990s. In women, prevalence of smoking increased in the 1970s and decreased slightly in the 1980s and 1990s. Body mass index showed a slight increase over the last decades, particularly in the second half of the 1980s. It is concluded that elevated major risk factors for coronary heart disease are still present in a large proportion of the Dutch population. To reduce the burden of chronic diseases in our aging society, influencing risk-factor levels in the general population is an important challenge for the years to come.

Key words. Trends—Cardiovascular disease risk factors—The Netherlands

Introduction

Cardiovascular diseases are still the most important cause of death in the Netherlands, even though mortality from them has declined during the last two decades [1]. Figures 1–3 show age-standardized mortality rates for cardio-vascular diseases (CVD, World Health Organization *International Classification of Diseases*, 9th rev., code 390–459), coronary heart disease (CHD, ICD-9 code 410–414), and cerebrovascular diseases (CVD, ICD-9 code 430–438). Mortality from cardiovascular diseases in men reached its peak in 1972. This coincides with the peak in CHD mortality, which is the largest

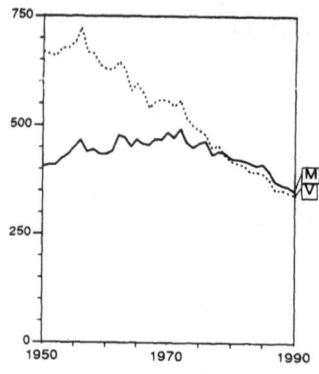

Fig. 1. Age-standardized mortality from cardio-vascular diseases (World Health Organization *International Classification of Diseases* codes 390–459) per 100 000 in the Netherlands since 1950. *M*, men; *V*, women

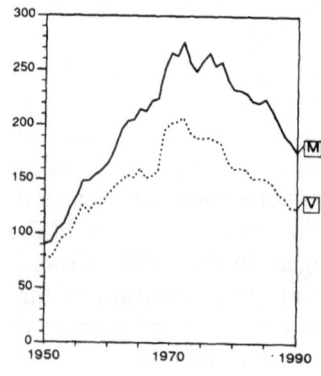

Fig. 2. Age-standardized mortality from coronary heart disease (World Health Organization *International Classification of Diseases* codes 410–414) per 100 000 in the Netherlands since 1950. *M*, men; *V*, women

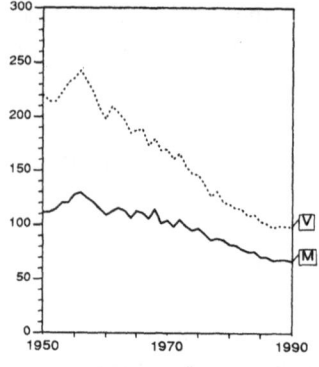

Fig. 3. Age-standardized mortality from cerebro-vascular diseases (World Health Organization *International Classification of Diseases* codes 430–438) per 100 000 in the Netherlands since 1950. *M*, men; *V*, women

contributor to total CVD mortality in men. Between 1972 and 1990, age-adjusted CHD mortality decreased by 29% in men and 38% in women. Mortality from cerebrovascular diseases started to decline in 1956, and since has declined by 49% in men and 59% in women.

The extent to which these changes can be attributed to primary prevention or to improved health care is not known. In this context, it is of interest to know what happened with the levels of the major CVD risk factors in the general population during the last decades. With respect to public health it is also important to get insight into the levels of the risk factors. To examine long-term trends in risk-factor levels, it is extremely important that measurements be performed in a strictly standardized way and in a well-defined study population over a long period of time. In the Netherlands, three screening projects can be used to establish trends in biological risk factors for CHD. These projects have been carried out consecutively in the periods 1974–1980, 1981–1986, and 1987–1991. The project carried out most recently will be used to describe current levels of CHD risk factors in the Netherlands. For smoking, data on a broad age range are available from surveys carried out by the National Foundation on Smoking and Public Health.

Methods

Study Populations

Consultation Bureau Project (CB-Project), 1974–1980. In 1972 a pilot study was carried out to examine if the network of consultation bureaus that existed in the Netherlands for screening of tuberculosis could be used for screening of cardiovascular disease risk factors. From October 1974 onward, a standardized protocol was used. The project started in the consultation bureaus in Doetinchem, a small town in a rural area in the eastern part of the country with about 40 000 inhabitants, and Tilburg, a town in the southwest with about 150 000 inhabitants. In 1976, three other cities were added to the study: Amsterdam, the capital city in the western part of the country with about 700 000 inhabitants, Leiden in the west, and Maastricht in the south, both with about 100 000 inhabitants. A total of 30 000 men and women aged 37–43 years was examined during this study period. The response rate was about 70%. The examination included measurement of blood pressure, weight, and height. A nonfasting blood sample was taken for the determination of total cholesterol. All subjects completed a questionnaire requesting information about smoking habits, cardiovascular complaints, family history of premature cardiovascular mortality, physical activity, and history of hypertension and diabetes.

Risk Factor Project on Cardiovascular Diseases (RIFOH-Project), 1981–1986. In 1981 the study protocol was changed in an attempt to make the study more cost-effective. The questionnaire was shortened, and the study focused mainly on the three major risk factors for CVD: smoking, blood pressure, and total cholesterol. Also, height and weight were measured. It was decided to examine only men because they were at higher risk for cardiovascular diseases than women. The study was aimed at relatively young men (around age 35) to be able to start primary prevention in high-risk adults at a young age. The project was carried out in the same five towns in which the CB-Project had taken place. The response rate was about 65%. From July 1981 to October 1986, a total of about 80000 men aged 33–37 years was examined.

Monitoring Project on Cardiovascular Disease Risk Factors (CVD Monitoring Project), 1987–1991. In 1987 the study protocol was changed. It was decided that it was necessary to have detailed information on CVD risk factors in the general population and a broader age range. Therefore, the age range was extended to 20–59 years, and again both men and women were examined. Each year a new random sample of men and women aged 20–59 was obtained for this project from the municipal registries. The questionnaire was extended to a large number of lifestyle factors, and three nonfasting blood samples were taken. Part of the blood was used for determination of total and HDL cholesterol; the remainder was stored at −20°C for future research. Height and weight were measured, and blood pressure was measured twice. Due to financial constraints, the project could not be continued in all five study centers, but only in Amsterdam, Doetinchem, and Maastricht. The response rate was about 50% in men and 57% in women. Between 1987 and 1991, a total of 36000 men and women aged 20–59 years was examined [2].

With respect to smoking habits, data in a broad age range are available from nationwide surveys, since 1958 on age groups 15 years and older [3,4]. Based on these surveys, yearly prevalence figures by age and gender are published by the Dutch Foundation on Smoking and Health. These publications were used to describe long-term trends qualitatively, while data of the CB, RIFOH, and CVD Monitoring Projects were used to describe smoking habits in a more detailed way (e.g., ex- and never-smoking, average daily consumption, and starting age of cigarette smoking).

Measurements

Total Cholesterol. During the entire period 1974–1991, total cholesterol was determined in the same laboratory, the Central Clinical Chemistry Laboratory of the University Hospital Dijkzigt in Rotterdam. This laboratory participates in the standardization program of the World Health Organization (WHO) through the WHO Regional Lipid Center for Europe in Prague, Czechoslovakia, and the Centers for Disease Control (CDC) in Atlanta, USA [5]. It is the Lipid Reference Laboratory for standardized cholesterol determinations in the Netherlands and also serves as an international member of the Cholesterol Reference Method Laboratories Network in the United States. In the CB-Project, total cholesterol was determined using a direct Liebermann–Burchard method [6], while in the RIFOH-Project and CVD Monitoring Project an enzymatic method was used [7]. Based on a comparison study in which over 5000 samples were analyzed with both methods, all values were converted to enzymatic values [8]. During the entire study period, the quality standards for certified laboratories of the WHO, as adopted by the CDC, were met, ensuring that the measurement of cholesterol concentration differed no more than 5% from the true level. However, a small laboratory drift, unimportant for clinical practice, can be disturbing for the analysis of trends. Therefore the internal quality control data of the laboratory were also analyzed to detect possible small changes over time. In both the CB-Project and the RIFOH-Project, there were periods in which the laboratory showed a small "drift," and in that case the cholesterol measurements during that period were corrected for this drift [8]. No laboratory drift was observed from 1987–1991. Hypercholesterolemia was defined as a total cholesterol level of 6.5 mmol/l (251 mg/dl) or more [9].

Blood Pressure. Blood pressure was measured in the left arm with a random zero sphygmomanometer, with the subject in sitting position. All measurements were carried out by trained technicians. Systolic blood pressure was recorded at the appearance of sounds (first-phase Korotkoff) and diastolic blood pressure at the disappearance of sounds (fifth-phase Korotkoff). In the CB-Project and the RIFOH-Project, a single blood pressure measurement was taken, and a cuff size 12×23 cm was used. In the CVD Monitoring Project blood pressure was measured twice, and if necessary a larger (15×33 cm) or smaller (9×18 cm) cuff was used. In the analysis, the mean of the two blood pressure readings was used for the CVD Monitoring Project. Hypertension was defined according to the criteria of the WHO: systolic ≥ 160 and/or diastolic ≥ 95 mmHg and/or use of antihypertensive medication [10]. The percentage of treated hypertensives is the proportion of those with hypertension who received treatment.

Smoking. Data on the smoking prevalence from the Dutch Foundation on Smoking and Public Health and from the CB/RIFOH projects are based upon the question, "Do you smoke?" Prevalence figures thus include cigarette, cigar, and pipe smokers. In the CB/RIFOH projects, an additional question was asked allowing to distinguish cigarette, cigar, or pipe smoking. The prevalence of cigarette smoking among men in the CB/RIFOH projects was about 5%–10% lower than the prevalence of all types of smoking. Prevalence figures from the Monitoring Project on Cardiovascular Disease Risk Factors are based on the questions, "Did you ever smoke cigarettes?," "Do you currently smoke cigarettes?," "How many cigarettes do you smoke per day?," and "At what age did you start to smoke cigarettes?"

Body Mass Index. Height was measured to the nearest 0.5 cm with a wall-mounted stadiometer, while the subject stood upright against the wall with the feet at a 45° angle. Weight was measured to the nearest 0.1 kg, with the respondent wearing indoor clothing, after taking off shoes and emptying pockets. Body mass index was calculated as weight $(kg)/height^2(m)$. Obesity was defined as a body mass index of 30 or more.

Statistical Methods

Analyses were carried out in all three projects using time (months) as the independent variable and risk-factor levels as the dependent variable. Linear regression analysis was used to describe changes over time. In the CB-Project, the change in cholesterol and blood pressure over time showed a U-shaped curve. Therefore two regression lines were fitted and the breakpoint in the line was determined by optimizing the explained variance [11].

In the CB-Project and RIFOH-Project (where the age range was quite small), adjustments for age were done on an individual basis. Based on regression equations for the relation between age and the risk-factor level, the risk-factor level for each person was extrapolated to age 40 (CB-Project) or age 35 (RIFOH-Project). For the CVD Monitoring Project (in which the age range was much broader), data were age-standardized to the age distribution of the general population aged 20–59 years in 1990. In the CB- and RIFOH-Project analyses, dummy variables were included for towns because the number of persons examined in each town differed from year to year, and risk-factor levels were slightly different between the towns. In the CVD Monitoring Project, no adjustment for town was necessary because numbers for the three towns were about equal.

For the analysis of trends in total cholesterol, the quality control data of the laboratory were analyzed to detect a possible "drift" (see "Materials and Methods"). Cholesterol values of the CB-Project and RIFOH-Project were corrected for laboratory "drift"; for the CVD Monitoring Project no adjustments were necessary. For trends in blood pressure, adjustments were made for the technician who had measured the blood pressure because analyses showed some differences in average blood pressure measured by different technicians.

Results

Below, results are described for the risk factors cholesterol, blood pressure, smoking, and body mass index. For each risk factor, first the levels are described, based on the CVD Monitoring Project. These data apply to men and women aged 20–59 years in the period 1987–1991. Secondly, changes in the risk factors that have taken place in the last two decades (1974–1991) are described, based on the three projects described in the "Materials and Methods" section. Because the age ranges of the populations studied in these projects are different, changes are described separately for each study period.

Total Cholesterol

In men, cholesterol levels and prevalence of hypercholesterolemia increase strongly until about age 40, after which the age increase levels off (Table 1).

Table 1. Total cholesterol (mmol/l[a]) by age and gender: mean, standard deviation, and prevalence of hypercholesterolemia (total cholesterol ≥ 6.5 mmol/l (≥ 251 mg/dl)). Monitoring Project on Cardiovascular Disease Risk Factors, 1987–1991, the Netherlands.

Age category	Men				Women			
	Number	Mean	SD	% ≥ 6.5 mmol/l	Number	Mean	SD	% ≥ 6.5 mmol/l
20–24	1336	4.47	0.82	1.6	1677	4.83	0.86	3.9
25–29	1755	4.95	0.96	6.7	1899	4.89	0.88	4.0
30–34	2170	5.21	1.02	10.5	2330	4.92	0.88	5.1
35–39	2290	5.48	1.09	16.6	2621	5.12	0.93	7.0
40–44	2480	5.78	1.12	23.0	2644	5.34	0.94	10.7
45–49	2405	5.89	1.08	26.0	2553	5.66	1.01	18.0
50–54	2328	5.99	1.08	29.5	2629	6.10	1.10	32.6
55–59	2290	6.00	1.05	29.8	2595	6.39	1.16	42.9
20–59[b]	17054	5.39		16.2	18948	5.30		13.0

SD, standard deviation.
[a] 1 mmol/l = 38.67 mg/dl.
[b] Standardized to the age distribution of the general population aged 20–59 in the Netherlands in 1990.

Mean levels in the youngest age group are around 4.5 mmol/l (174 mg/dl) compared with 6.0 mmol/l (232 mg/dl) in the oldest age group. The prevalence of hypercholesterolemia (total cholesterol ≥ 6.5 mmol/l, ≥ 251 mg/dl) increases from about 2% in the youngest to 30% in the oldest age group. In women, the increase is especially strong from age 40 onward, partly due to the occurrence of menopause (Table 1). In the youngest age groups average total cholesterol levels are around 4.8 mmol/l (186 mg/dl), while in the oldest age group total cholesterol levels have increased to 6.4 mmol/l (247 mg/dl). Likewise, the prevalence of hypercholesterolemia increased from about 4% to about 43%.

Between 1974 and 1980 a decrease followed by an increase in total cholesterol levels was observed in men and women aged 37–43 years (Fig. 4). This resulted in a net decrease over the total study period of 0.07 mmol/l (3 mg/dl) in men and 0.03 mmol/l (1 mg/dl) in women [8]. The prevalence of hypercholesterolemia showed a net decline of about 3 percentage points in men and 2 percentage points in women. From 1981–1986, total cholesterol declined by 0.2 mmol/l (8 mg/dl) in men aged 33–37 years (Fig. 5). Accordingly, the prevalence of hypercholesterolemia declined by about 5.5 percentage points [8]. Over the period 1987–1991, total cholesterol levels and the prevalence of hypercholesterolemia were stable in men and women, while in 1991 a decrease was observed of about 0.1 mmol/l (4 mg/dl) in total cholesterol levels (Fig. 6) and of about 2.5 percentage points in men and 1.5 percentage points in women in the prevalence of hypercholesterolemia.

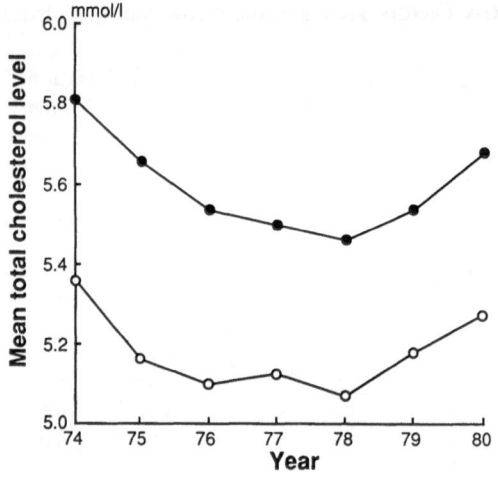

Fig. 4. Mean total cholesterol level per year in men (*solid circles*) and women (*open circles*) aged 40 (±3) years in the period 1974–1980. Consultation Bureau Project, the Netherlands

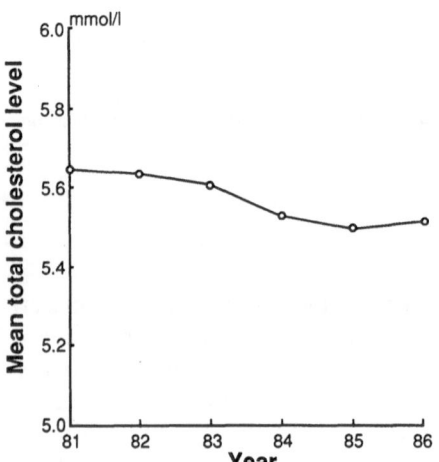

Fig. 5. Mean total cholesterol level per year in men aged 35 (±2) years in the period 1980–1986. Risk Factor Project on Cardiovascular Diseases, the Netherlands

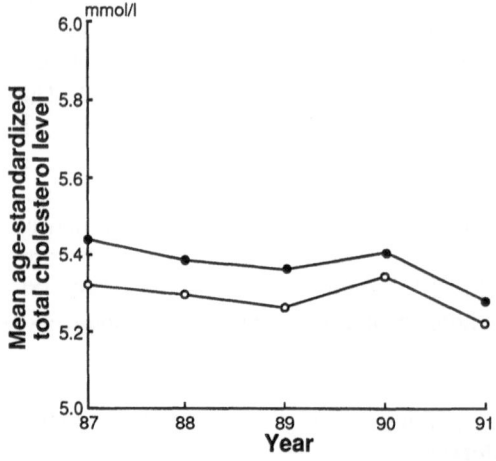

Fig. 6. Mean age-standardized total cholesterol level per year in men (*solid circles*) and women (*open circles*) aged 20–59 years. Monitoring Project on Cardiovascular Disease Risk Factors, 1987–1991, the Netherlands

Blood Pressure

For men and women, both systolic and diastolic blood pressure increased with age after about age 40 (Tables 2 and 3). In all 5-year age categories, systolic and diastolic blood pressure were higher in men than in women. The prevalence of hypertension also increased with age in both men and women. The prevalence of hypertension was higher for men than for women except in the two oldest age categories, where the prevalence in both sexes was about the same. In all 5-year age categories, a higher percentage of women was treated for hypertension than men (Tables 2 and 3).

In the period 1974–1980, average systolic blood pressure increased by 2 mmHg in men aged 37–43 years, while systolic blood pressure did not change in women during that period. Average diastolic blood pressure increased by

Table 2. Mean blood pressure (mmHg) and standard deviation, prevalence of hypertension, and percentage of treated hypertensives for men by age categories.

Age category	Number	Mean systolic blood pressure	SD	Mean diastolic blood pressure	SD	% Hypertension	% Treated hypertensives
20–24	1 338	121.3	11.5	72.6	8.6	1.2	6.3
25–29	1 758	121.6	11.7	74.0	8.7	2.2	12.8
30–34	2 175	121.4	11.8	75.7	9.1	2.8	19.4
35–39	2 295	121.2	12.7	77.0	9.8	5.8	22.4
40–44	2 478	122.9	13.1	79.2	9.7	8.6	33.5
45–49	2 409	124.5	14.8	80.4	10.3	12.5	37.5
50–54	2 329	127.7	16.0	81.1	10.3	16.1	47.5
55–59	2 295	130.6	17.5	81.4	10.2	21.7	55.3
20–59[a]	17 077	123.3		77.1		7.5	26.3

[a] Standardized to age distribution of the general population aged 20–59 years in the Netherlands in 1990.

Table 3. Mean blood pressure (mmHg) and standard deviation, prevalence of hypertension, and percentage of treated hypertensives for women by age categories.

Age category	Number	Mean systolic blood pressure	SD	Mean diastolic blood pressure	SD	% Hypertension	% Treated hypertensives
20–24	1 695	111.5	10.4	69.9	8.4	0.6	9.1
25–29	1 907	110.9	10.8	70.3	8.7	1.3	36.0
30–34	2 332	110.6	11.2	70.6	8.8	1.4	50.0
35–39	2 630	111.9	12.0	72.5	9.1	2.7	50.0
40–44	2 659	115.0	13.7	74.3	9.5	5.0	45.1
45–49	2 567	118.6	16.1	76.3	10.1	9.7	57.0
50–54	2 650	123.3	16.9	78.4	10.3	15.8	63.6
55–59	2 597	126.9	17.4	79.2	10.4	21.8	68.1
20–59[a]	19 037	114.7		73.3		5.9	44.7

[a] Standardized to age distribution of the general population aged 20–59 years in the Netherlands in 1990.

4 mmHg in men and 2 mmHg in women. The prevalence of hypertension in men increased from 12.7% in 1974 to 17.8% in 1980, while in women, it was 8.5% and did not change between 1974–1980 [12] (Fig. 7). Treatment of hypertensive men increased from 8% in 1974 to 21% in 1980. Treatment of hypertensive women did not change and amounted to 28%. Between 1981 and 1986, average systolic blood pressure did not change in men aged 33–37 years, while average diastolic blood pressure decreased by 4 mmHg (Fig. 8). The prevalence of hypertension did not change and amounted to 9.6%. Treatment of hypertensive men increased from 9% in 1981 to 13% in 1986 [13]. Between 1987 and 1991, changes in systolic and diastolic blood pressure were minor in both men and women aged 20–59 years (Fig. 9). In this period, the prevalence of hypertension did not change in men and women. Treatment of hypertensive men decreased from 44% in 1987 to 34% in 1991, and treatment of hypertensive women decreased from 60% to 49% [13].

Smoking

The overall prevalence of smoking in men and women (aged 15 years and older) was 38% and 31%, respectively, in 1993 [4]. Table 4 shows the age-specific prevalence of smoking in men and women aged 20–59 years between 1987 and 1991 as observed in the Monitoring Project on Cardiovascular Disease Risk Factors [8]. The prevalence of smoking was highest in men and women aged 30–39 years. The prevalence of quitting in men strongly increased with age, from 26% in the youngest to 51% in the oldest. In women, the prevalence of quitting increased with age, from 26% in the youngest women to 39% in women 40–49 years old. In the oldest women, the prevalence of quitting was 31%.

Table 4. Smoking prevalence by age and gender. Monitoring Project on Cardiovascular Disease Risk Factors, 1987–1991, The Netherlands.

Age category	Men		Women	
	Number	Percent	Number	Percent
20–24	1336	35.7	1723	36.2
25–29	1757	39.9	2006	40.7
30–34	2176	43.8	2453	44.6
35–39	2292	43.0	2674	43.5
40–44	2476	40.9	2660	41.4
45–49	2409	40.4	2565	37.1
50–54	2326	38.4	2648	35.3
55–59	2291	38.4	2259	33.3
20–59[a]	17066	40.2	19326	39.6

[a] Standardized to age distribution of the general population aged 20–59 in the Netherlands in 1990.

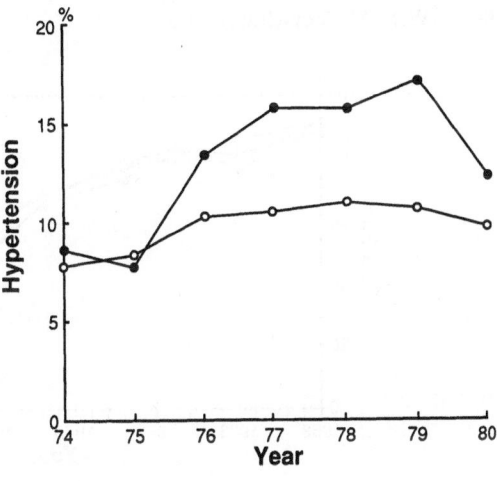

Fig. 7. Prevalence of hypertension in 40(±3)-year-old men (*solid circles*) and women (*open circles*) in the period 1974–1980. Consultation Bureau Project, the Netherlands

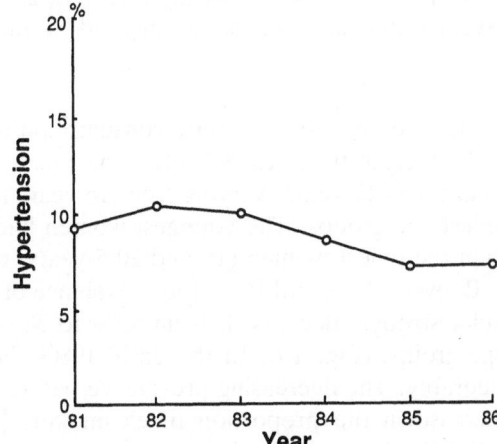

Fig. 8. Prevalence of hypertension in 35(±2)-year-old men in the period 1981–1986. Risk Factor-Project on Cardiovascular Diseases, the Netherlands

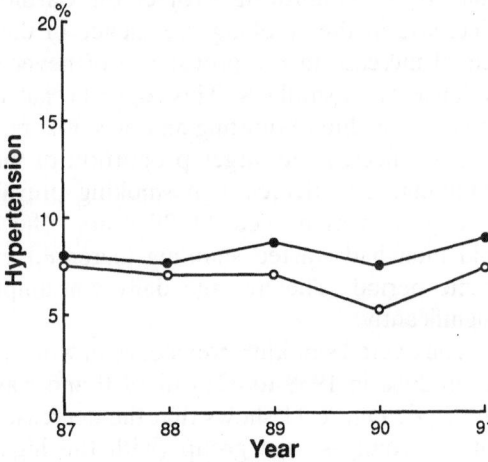

Fig. 9. Prevalence of hypertension in men (*solid circles*) and women (*open circles*) aged 20–59 years in the period 1987–1991. Monitoring Project on Cardiovascular Disease Risk Factors, the Netherlands

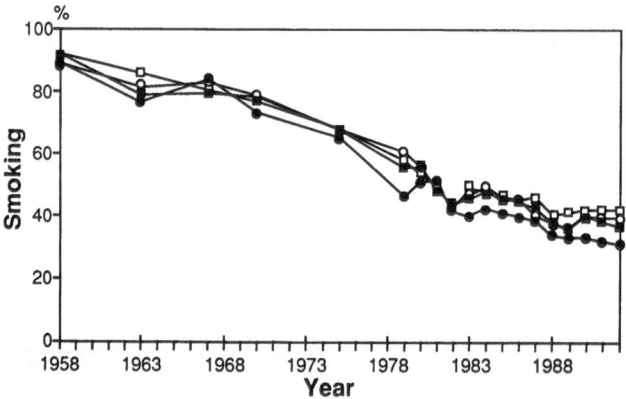

Fig. 10. Prevalence of smoking in men for different age groups 20–34 (*solid squares*), 35–49 (*open squares*), 50–64 (*open circles*), and 65+ (*solid circles*) between 1958 and 1992. Dutch Foundation on Smoking and Health 1958–1992

The average daily cigarette consumption in men and women smokers was 16 and 15 cigarettes, respectively. The mean age at which men had started to smoke was 17 years, varying from 16 years in the youngest to 17.5 years in the oldest age groups. The youngest women had started smoking at an earlier age than the oldest women (16 and 20.5 years, respectively).

Between 1958 and 1992, the prevalence of smoking in men aged 15 years and older strongly decreased, from 90% to 38% [4]. The decrease was seen in all age groups (Fig. 10). In the early 1980s, however, the decrease slowed considerably. The decreasing prevalence before 1980 was accompanied by a strong increase in the proportion of ex-smokers [3]. During the period 1981–1986 (RIFOH-Project), the increase in the percentage of never-smokers was generally greater than the increase in the percentage of ex-smokers. Between 1987 and 1991 (Monitoring Project on Cardiovascular Disease Risk Factors), a decrease in the smoking prevalence of 0.6% per year was observed, with an equal increase in the prevalence of never-smokers and no change in the prevalence of ex-smokers. This suggests that the decrease in the 1960s and 1970s was largely due to quitting among smokers, whereas the smaller decrease in the 1980s reflected the larger proportion of men who never took up the habit of smoking. The decrease in smoking prevalence between 1987 and 1991 was strongest in men aged 20–29 years. The age at which these 20- to 29-year-old men had started smoking increased by approximately 1 year during the same period. The average daily consumption of cigarettes has not changed significantly.

The overall smoking prevalence in women (aged 15 years and older) increased from 29% in 1958 to 42% in 1970 and was followed by a decrease to 31% in 1992 [4]. Figure 11 shows that the decrease in smoking prevalence was greatest in the youngest age group (with the highest smoking prevalence). Between

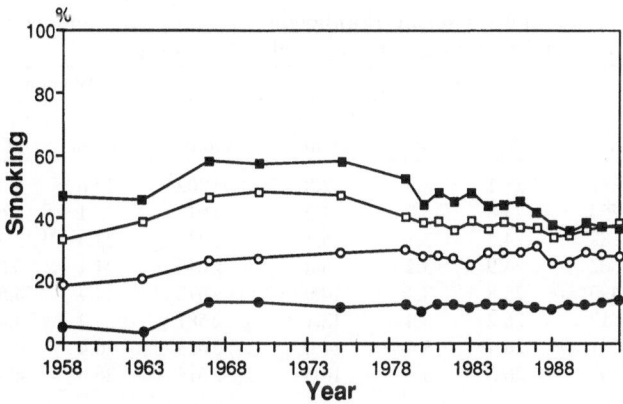

Fig. 11. Prevalence of smoking in women for different age groups 20–34 (*solid squares*), 35–49 (*open squares*), 50–64 (*open circles*), and 65+ (*solid circles*) between 1958 and 1992. Dutch Foundation on Smoking and Health 1958–1992

1958 and 1982, the prevalence of ex-smokers increased, whereas the prevalence of never-smokers decreased until 1972 and then remained approximately stable [3]. Data from the Monitoring Project on Cardiovascular Disease Risk Factors showed an overall decrease of smoking prevalence of 0.8 percentage points per year between 1987 and 1991. The decrease was mainly due to a decrease of 1.9 percentage points per year in 20- to 29-year-old women. The decrease was accompanied by a similar increase in the prevalence of never-smokers in this age group. During the same period, the average daily consumption in women decreased slightly (one cigarette over the total period) in younger women (20–29 years). No changes were observed in older women. The age at which smokers had started smoking decreased in women aged 30 years and older, but not in women under 30 years of age.

Body Mass Index

Cross-sectionally in both men and women, mean body mass index increased with age. In men an average difference of about $3 \, kg/m^2$ was observed between the age group 45–49 years and the age group 20–24 years. After age 45, the mean body mass index remained relatively stable with advancing age (Table 5). In women, the increase of average BMI with age continued throughout all age categories studied. Average BMI in women was lower compared to men in all age groups except in those aged 55–59 years. The prevalence of obesity (BMI $> 30 \, kg/m^2$) was higher in women in all age groups, which could be explained by the larger variance in BMI in women across all ages (Table 5).

Blokstra and Kromhout reported that in the period 1974–1980, the average BMI increased by about $0.5 \, kg/m^2$ in men aged 37–43 years, whereas in women no significant trend was observed [14]. The percentage of obese men

Table 5. Body mass index (weight (kg)/height $(m)^2$) by age and gender: means, standard deviations, and percentage of overweight ($\geq 30 \, kg/m^2$).

Age category	Men				Women			
	Number	Mean	SD	% $\geq$ 30 kg/m^2	Number	Mean	SD	% $\geq$ 30 kg/m^2
20–24	1341	23.1	2.9	2.8	1702	22.6	3.3	3.2
25–29	1760	23.8	3.2	4.2	1913	23.1	3.6	4.7
30–34	2182	24.5	3.1	5.1	2340	23.4	3.7	5.7
35–39	2302	24.9	3.2	5.8	2645	24.1	3.8	7.3
40–44	2490	25.8	3.4	10.0	2672	24.7	4.0	9.0
45–49	2417	26.2	3.4	12.1	2581	25.7	4.4	15.2
50–54	2341	26.4	3.4	14.0	2663	26.4	4.3	16.6
55–59	2303	26.3	3.2	10.5	2614	26.8	4.3	18.9
20–59[a]	17136	24.9		7.4	19130	24.3		9.0

[a] Standardized to age distribution of the general population aged 20–59 in the Netherlands in 1990.

and women did not change significantly over this period. In the period 1981–1986, there was no change in either the average BMI or the prevalence of obesity in men aged 33–37 years [14]. Preliminary analysis of the data obtained in the period 1987–1991 suggested that average BMI did not increase significantly when corrected for age. Over this period, the level of education among participants in the project increased significantly. When additional corrections were made for educational level there was a significant linear increase in BMI, which amounted to an increase of about $0.2 \, kg/m^2$ in men and $0.3 \, kg/m^2$ in women over the 5-year period. The prevalence of obesity increased in both men and women by about 2 percentage points when corrected for age and educational level.

Discussion

Elevated major risk factors for coronary heart disease are still present in a large proportion of the Dutch population. Available data on cholesterol levels during the last decades concern different age groups. Especially the projects carried out between 1974–1986 involve only a limited age range. During 1974–1980 almost no net decrease was observed in blood cholesterol, while in the early 1980s a decrease was observed in relatively young adult men. With data from the Zutphen Study, we investigated if the change in young men was also observed in middle-aged men. It was shown that men aged 40–59 years in 1985 had higher levels than men aged 40–59 years in 1960 [15]. From the Zutphen Study, data on men aged 65–69 in 1970, 1977–1978, and 1985 were also available. In these data, a U-shaped relation between time and total cholesterol was also observed. Therefore it was concluded that the change in relatively young men was not generalizable to other age groups. Data collected from 1987–1991 suggest a decrease in the last year. The future will have to tell if this decrease is persistent. Given the relatively high total cholesterol level in the Netherlands, we conclude that over the last decades, the changes in total cholesterol level in men and women in the Netherlands have been small, with the exception of a decline of 0.2 mmol/l in relatively young adult men during the early 1980s. Unfortunately, no data for women are available for the early 1980s.

At the beginning of the 1960s, cholesterol levels in the Netherlands were comparable to those in the United States [16]. Within Europe a strong north-south gradient was present at that time, with the highest levels in Scandinavian countries, intermediate levels in mid-European countries such as the Netherlands, and lowest levels in the Mediterranean countries. Since that time, cholesterol levels in the United States and Scandinavian countries have decreased, while cholesterol levels in Mediterranean countries, for example, Italy, have increased. At present, cholesterol levels in the Netherlands are higher than those in the United States, are comparable to levels in Italy, but are still somewhat lower than those in the Scandinavian countries [17]. The relatively high total cholesterol level in the Netherlands can partly be explained by the food consumption pattern of the Dutch, characterized by intake of a high percentage of saturated fat. The past decades on average at least 40% of energy was derived from fat (of which about 16 energy percent is saturated fat). In the past few years, special campaigns have been carried out to decrease fat intake, and there are indications that the total fat intake and saturated fat intake may be declining.

It is difficult to compare mean levels of blood pressure between different study periods because of differences in blood pressure measurements and differences in age of the study population. In contrast to levels, however, trends in the prevalence and treatment of hypertension from different study periods can be compared. In all study periods, no decrease in the prevalence of hypertension has been observed. In the period between 1974 and 1986 treatment of hypertensive men increased, while between 1987 and 1991 treatment of hypertensive men decreased. Treatment of hypertensive women did not change between 1974 and 1980, while during 1987–1991 treatment of hypertensive women decreased. Thus, from 1987 onward a decrease in treatment of hypertension was observed in both men and women. The decrease in treatment can be due to the fact that in the mid-1980s the usefulness of drug treatment for mild hypertension was heavily debated among general practitioners [18]. From that time onward the diagnosis of hypertension was based on several blood pressure measurements instead of just one [19]. This resulted in a reduction of the number of subjects treated for hypertension because only subjects with "real" high blood pressure were treated.

In the Netherlands a decrease in treatment of hypertension has been observed, while in other countries (e.g., United States, Italy, and Japan) such a decrease has not [20–23]. This can be due to the fact that, for instance in the

United States, the National High Blood Pressure Education Program had already started in 1972 [24]. From that time onward, physicians were trained to diagnose and treat hypertension according to guidelines. In the Netherlands, there is no such nationwide program.

Smoking is the risk factor that is most prevalent, since about 40% of men and women smoke. This figure is more or less the same in all age groups between age 20 and 59. Over the last 35 years, smoking prevalence has decreased in men. However, the decrease has slowed considerably since the early 1980s and has almost come to a standstill in the 1990s. In women, an increase in smoking prevalence was observed until the 1970s. This was followed by a decrease in the 1980s and 1990s. The recent decrease is largely due to decreasing smoking prevalence in the youngest women, whereas the prevalence in older women seems to have stabilized, as in men. The question therefore arises whether smoking prevalence is still changing for the better. To answer this question, we distinguish two causes of decrease in smoking prevalence: an increasing prevalence of ex-smokers and an increasing prevalence of never-smokers. Antismoking campaigns may encourage smokers to quit. Nevertheless, it is likely that a group of persistent smokers will remain. The slowing decline of smoking prevalence after 1980 in men and in women older than 30 years is possibly due to that phenomenon. The smoking prevalence several decades from now will be strongly determined by the smoking prevalence in currently young age groups (cohort effect). In that respect, the increasing prevalence of never-smokers in men and women aged 20–29 years and the increase in starting age that was observed in young men over the period 1987–1991, are encouraging. However, data from the Dutch Foundation on Smoking and Health show that smoking prevalence in men and women under 20 years of age has stabilized at a level of approximately 20% during the last few years. Without further decrease, the smoking prevalence may remain at that level for many decades to come.

Prevalence of obesity in the Netherlands seems to have slightly increased over the last decades in men and women, particularly in the second half of the 1980s when it increased about 2 percentage points. A similar increase was reported by the Dutch Central Bureau of Statistics, which based its conclusions on reported height and weight in the Dutch Health Interview Surveys 1981–1988 [25]. Also, other countries such as Denmark, Sweden, and the United Kingdom have reported increases in the prevalence of obesity during the 1980s [26–28].

Mortality statistics show that mortality rates for CHD in persons aged 30 years or older have declined in both men and women. However, for persons aged 50 and older, hospital admission rates have increased; for ages 30–49 years they have decreased [29]. This indicates that the reduction in older age strata is (partly) due to medical care, while in the younger age strata, an effect of primary prevention on mortality rates also plays a role.

Still, it remains difficult to estimate the contribution of primary prevention to the decline in coronary heart disease in the Netherlands because changes in risk-factor levels do not immediately lead to changes in mortality. The decline in smoking prevalence probably contributed most strongly to this decline in coronary heart disease mortality in men. It is less likely that changes in total cholesterol levels and blood pressure have contributed to this, because the available data do not indicate that major changes have taken place in levels of these risk factors. The decrease in mortality from cerebrovascular disease that started already in 1956 can be only partly due to increasing treatment of hypertension, since antihypertensive drugs were not widely used before 1970. These changes, however, took place long before monitoring data were available, and are therefore speculative.

Knowledge of risk factors and of mechanisms important in the etiology of coronary heart disease has increased considerably over the last decades and is still progressing. However, much less progress has been made in knowledge on how to influence risk-factor levels and lifestyle habits in the general population. To reduce the burden of chronic diseases in aging societies, this is an important challenge for the years to come.

References

1. Mortality according to cause of death, age and gender (A1-series) (in Dutch). Centraal Bureau voor de Statistiek, Voorburg, Netherlands
2. Verschuren WMM, Leer van EM, Blokstra A, Seidell JC, Smit HA, Bueno de Mesquita HB, Obermann-de Boer GL, Kromhout D (1993) Cardiovascular disease risk factors in the Netherlands. Neth J Cardiol 6:205–210
3. Van Reek J (1984) Smoking behaviour in the Netherlands and the United Kingdom: 1958–1982. Rev Epidemiol Sante Publ 32:383–390
4. Dutch Foundation on Smoking and Health (Stichting Volksgezondheid en Roken) (1993) Annual report 1992, The Hague, Netherlands
5. Myers GL, Cooper GR, Winn CL, Smith SJ (1989) The Center for Disease Control —National Heart, Lung, and Blood Institute Lipid Standardization Program. Clin Lab Med 9:105–135
6. Huang TC, Chen CP, Wefler V, Raftery A (1961) A stable reagent for the Liebermann-Burchard reaction: application to rapid serum cholesterol determination. Anal Chem 33:1405–1407
7. Katterman R, Jaworek D, Moller G (1984) Multicenter study of a new enzymatic method of cholesterol determination. J Clin Chem Clin Biochem 22:245–251
8. Verschuren WMM, Al M, Blokstra A, Boerma GJM, Kromhout D. Trend in serum total cholesterol level in 110 000 young adults in the Netherlands, 1974 to 1986. Am J Epidemiol 134:1290–1302
9. Anonymous (1992) Netherlands Cholesterol Consensus Update (in Dutch). Hart Bulletin [Suppl]23:9–21
10. World Health Organization (1985) Final report of the working group on risk and high blood pressure. An epidemiological approach to describing risk associated with blood pressure levels. Hypertension 7:457–468
11. Kleinbaum DG, Kupper LL, Muller KE (1988) Applied regression analysis and other multivariable methods. PWS-KENT Publishing, Boston, Mass., pp 265–279

12. Van Leer EM, Verschuren WMM, Kromhout D (1994) Trends in blood pressure and the prevalence and treatment of hypertension in young adults in the Netherlands, 1974–1986. Eur J Epidemiol 10:151–158

13. Van Leer EM, Seidell JC, Kromhout D (to be published) Levels and trends in blood pressure, prevalence and treatment of hypertension in 36 723 men and women aged 20–59 years in the Netherlands from 1987–1991. Am J Prev Med

14. Blokstra A, Kromhout D (1991) Trends in obesity in young adults in the Netherlands, 1974–1986. Int J Obes 15:513–521

15. Kromhout D, De Lezenne Coulander C, Obermann-de Boer GL, van Kampen-Donker M, Goddijn HE, Bloemberg BPM (1990) Changes in food and nutrient intake in middle-aged men from 1960 to 1985 (the Zutphen Study). Am J Clin Nutr 51:123–129

16. Keys A (1970) Coronary heart disease in seven countries. Circulation 41[Suppl I]:1–211

17. WHO (1989) The WHO MONICA Project: a worldwide monitoring system for cardiovascular diseases. World Health Statistics Annual

18. Boot CPM (1988) Is treatment of hypertension useful (in Dutch)? Medisch Contact 42:1311–1314

19. Binsbergen JJ van, Grundmeyer HGLM, Hoogen JPH van den (1991) Dutch general practitioners consensus on hypertension (in Dutch). Huisarts en Wetenschap 8:389–395

20. Green MS, Peled I (1992) Prevalence and control of hypertension in a large cohort of occupationally-active Israelis examined during 1985–1987: The Cordis Study. Int J Epidemiol 21:676–682

21. Burke GL, Sprafka JM, Folsom AR, Luepker RV, Norsted SW, Blackburn H (1989) Trends in CHD mortality, morbidity and risk factor levels from 1960 to 1986: The Minnesota Heart Survey. Int J Epidemiol 18[Suppl I]:S73–S81

22. The Research Group ATS-RF2-OB43 of the Italian National Research Council (1987) Time trends of some cardiovascular risk factors in Italy. Results from the Nine Communities Study. Am J Epidemiol 126:95–103

23. Ueshima H, Tatara K, Asakura S (1987) Declining mortality from ischemic heart disease and changes in coronary risk factors in Japan, 1956–1980. Am J Epidemiol 125:62–72

24. National Heart, Lung, and Blood Institute (1991) Fact book, fiscal year 1990. U.S. Department of Health and Human Services

25. Verweij GCG (1989) Gezondheidsenquetes. Ontwikkelingen in onder- en overgewicht, 1981–1988. Maandbericht Gezondheidsstatistiek 11:5–10

26. Price RA, Ness R, Sorensen TIA (1990) Changes in commingled body mass index distributions associated with secular trends in overweight among Danish young men. Int J Obes 14:411–419

27. Kukowska-Wolk A, Bergstrom R (1993) Trends in body mass index and prevalence of obesity in Swedish men 1980–1989. J Epidemiol Commun Health 47:103–108

28. Gregory J, Foster K, Tyler H, Wiseman M (1990) The dietary and nutritional survey of British adults. Office of Population Census and Surveys, Social Survey Division, Her Majesty's Stationery Office, London

29. Hoogendoorn D (1990) Some remarks about the present state of the epidemic with respect to acute myocardial infarction (in Dutch). Ned Tijdschr Geneeskd 134:592–595

Mortality and Risk-factor Trends in Minnesota: Minnesota Heart Studies

DAVID R. JACOBS, JR., J. MICHAEL SPRAFKA, PETER J. HANNAN,
CYNTHIA M. RIPSIN, PAUL G. MCGOVERN, and HENRY BLACKBURN

Summary. Recent trends in Minnesota mortality rates and coronary heart disease risk-factor levels were examined in data from the Minnesota Heart Health Program and state vital statistics. Trends in underlying causes of death were examined for all Minnesota deaths occurring between 1969 and 1991. Risk-factor levels were examined based on serial cross-sectional population-based surveys of 300–500 persons each in six communities during the 1980s. The results were as follows:

1. Mortality rates in Minnesota for all-causes and most specific causes during 1969–1991 generally declined in people below age 85, and were stable in people at age 85 and above.

2. Death rates declined for most cardiovascular causes, coronary heart disease, and most cancers other than lung, liver, brain, and prostate.

3. Death rates in people aged 55–74 years increased for late-stage coronary heart disease (arrhythmias and congestive heart failure) and for stroke, lung cancer, and chronic obstructive pulmonary disease; prostate, liver, and brain cancers; endocrine and metabolic diseases (excluding diabetes); AIDS; septicemia; and senile dementia.

4. Coronary heart disease risk-factor levels generally decreased through the 1980s, with the exception of body mass index. Slope of change in serum total cholesterol closely paralleled slope of change in Keys score applied to dietary survey data. The steady increase in body mass index and the plateau in the level of leisure time physical activity, together with the lack of change in dietary caloric intake, suggest that work- and transportation-related physical activity decreased.

With a few exceptions, cause-specific mortality rates decreased in Minnesota in an era of cardiovascular risk-factor decline. Continued risk-factor reduction is clearly warranted, along with continued surveillance of trends in mortality, morbidity, and risk factors.

Key words. Cardiovascular risk factors—Cause-specific mortality—Surveillance

Introduction

Coronary heart disease (CHD) mortality in the U.S. and in Minnesota has declined steadily since the late 1960s. There is much evidence that the decline is the result of combined effects of improvement in medical care and in population levels of cardiovascular disease (CVD) risk factors. The relative contribution of these components to the observed decline is unknown, but one report estimated that primary prevention (i.e., smoking prevention, hypertension control, reduction of blood cholesterol level) explained about two-thirds of the decline, suggesting that risk-factor changes play a major role in observed CHD mortality patterns [1]. A 1994 PhD thesis modeled the decline in CHD deaths in relation to observed morbidity and risk-factor change, and attributed more than half the observed CHD decline in Minnesota to risk-factor changes [2].

Numerous studies have documented favorable risk-factor changes during the period of the 1970s and 1980s. Comparisons between the first (1971–1974) and second (1976–1980) National Health and Nutrition Examination Surveys suggest a decline in blood pressure and serum total cholesterol levels among national samples [3,4]. A recent report documents the continuing decline in serum total cholesterol level among U.S. adults between 1980 and 1990 [5]. Data from seven National Health Interview Surveys (1974–1985) indicate favorable (though not equal) declines across all race-gender groups in the prevalence and initiation of cigarette smoking [6].

Earlier reports from surveys and studies in Minnesota are consistent with these observations and indicate declines in smoking and blood cholesterol, with increases in blood pressure treatment and in physical activity in a random cohort of Twin Cities men first examined in 1966, and followed in 1975 [7]. The Minnesota Heart Study (MHS) has reported declines in the prevalence of cigarette smoking and decreases in serum total cholesterol and systolic and diastolic blood pressure levels, first between 1973 and 1980 (compared with a Lipid Research Clinics survey) [8], and later between 1980 and 1985 population surveys [9]. Leisure time physical activity (LTPA) has been monitored in the Twin Cities and the Upper Midwest using a single questionnaire, starting with the U.S. Railroad Study in 1957–1960. LTPA increased over a 30-year period [10]. However, body mass index has increased over time, together with the long-term increase in LTPA, suggesting that activity expended at work and getting to and from work has declined.

Mortality rates have generally declined. Total and coronary heart disease mortality rates have declined consistently, with little compensatory increase in non-CVD deaths. Stroke mortality rates declined rapidly through the 1970s, less rapidly in the 1980s, and recently appear to be on a plateau.

The Minnesota Heart Health Program (MHHP) conducted mortality, morbidity, and risk-factor surveillance throughout the 1980s. Its findings on trends are consistent with the findings of the MHS. In this chapter we present Minnesota mortality findings in greater detail and report for the first time findings on risk-factor trends from the MHHP. The risk-factor findings presented here occurred in the latter half of the period of mortality observation, so it is not possible to synchronize the two sets of findings presented in this paper. Nevertheless, the findings add to the evidence that, with the exception of selected causes of death, mortality change has been generally favorable in an era of continuing favorable risk-factor change in the population.

Methods

Mortality analyses are based on ICD (World Health Organization, *International Classification of Diseases*) coding of underlying cause of death using all death certificates in Minnesota (about 40 000 per year) for deaths occurring between 1969 and 1991. Average annual death rates were computed for four age groups and five time periods: 1969–1973, 1974–1978, 1979–1983, 1984–1988, and for the shorter time window 1989–1991. Variances of the mortality rates were computed separately for each cause of death from the mean square error of the sequence of 20 annual rates (1969–1988), after removal of quartic polynomial trends. As a summary measure of change, we computed the absolute and percent change in average annual death rate during 1984–1988 compared to the rate during 1968–1973. For each cause of death and age-sex group, we examined the entire sequence of average annual death rates (through 1989–1991) and the summary change measure, and reported as increasing or decreasing those changes in age-sex-disease specific rates which were statistically significant ($P < 0.05$). Virtually all such changes were found to be highly statistically significant. Mortality rate tables were summarized as they were too voluminous to present in their entirety.

Risk-factor trends were computed from serial cross-sectional surveys in six Midwestern communities of the Minnesota Heart Health Program (MHHP). Standardized probability surveys were done annually for 6 years during the 1980s in Mankato and Winona; 7 years in Fargo Moorhead and Sioux Falls; and 8 years in Bloomington and Roseville. Surveys were done in three stages (home enumeration, home interview, and clinic visit) and consistently had close to an overall 88% response rate at the home interview and 79% at the clinic. Nonrespondents tended to have lower socioeconomic status and to be smokers. Surveys included 300–500 people each. Periodic resurveys of baseline cohorts were also carried out by MHHP, but did not enter these analyses. MHHP mounted an education and intervention program in three of the communities, with the purpose of affecting populationwide changes in cardiovascular risk factors [11,12]. Because intervention effects in MHHP were small, data from educated and control communities were combined in this study of risk factor trends. Allowance was made for the fact that not all cities were surveyed in each calendar year, as follows: Mean levels or prevalences were computed within 48 community-age-sex groups for each risk factor, for each calendar year of observation. Home interview data were used for current smoking and clinic data for all other variables. The average of two blood pressures was used, measured seated after a 5-min rest, using a random zero sphygmomanometer. Blood serum was obtained by venipuncture and serum total cholesterol measured in the Minnesota Lipid Research Clinics laboratory. Height and weight were measured in stocking feet and light clothing. In half the sample, dietary data were obtained using a 24-h recall; in the other half, a detailed physical activity assessment was carried out using the Minnesota Leisure Time Physical Activity Questionnaire. Keys score, change in which closely parallels changes in serum total cholesterol, was computed from the 24-h dietary recall data as: $1.26 \times (2S - P) + 1.5/Z$, where S is the percent of dietary calories from lauric, myristic, and palmitic acids; P is the percent of calories from polyunsaturated fats; and Z is dietary cholesterol (mg/1000 Kcal).

The data were pooled in a regression model using SAS PROC MIXED, with calendar years represented as dummy variables and age, sex, and community as covariates. Calendar year was a repeated factor. Data were weighted by survey sample size. For each variable, this procedure resulted in a series of ten predicted levels (for 1981–1990) evaluated at an average level for community, age, and sex. Models were run separately by gender, with and without terms for interaction between time trend and age group. Additional models for each risk factor listed in Table 3 represented age and time trend as linear terms. References to baseline in this paper are to a summary of 1981–1984 data in each community.

Results

Changes in Mortality Rates

Table 1 and Fig. 1 show that total mortality rates declined between 1969 and 1988 in Minnesota for ages 35–54, 55–74, and 75–84. The percent decline was greatest in the younger age group, while the absolute decline was greatest in those 75–84 years old. These declines in total death rates imply that death is delayed in people as old as 84 years, yet even the rate of death for those over 85 declined slightly in women and was stable in men. Rates of total deaths continued to decline from 1989–1991. Declines in CVD mortality rate were more pronounced and consistent than those in total deaths, occurring even among men and women aged more than 85 years. Small increases in cancer mortality rates were seen in ages 55 and greater in both genders. Noncardiovascular, noncancer death rates were stable up to age 74; they increased slightly in those aged 75–84, and increased markedly in those greater than age 85.

Table 2 shows specific causes of death in which rates increased or declined. Declines in CHD death rates in each age group (about 45%) and in total stroke death rates (about 55%) were more pronounced than the corresponding decline

Table 1. Reports of underlying cause of death in Minnesota (rates per 100 000 population).

	Age at death (years)	Death rate, 1969–1973	Change through 1984–1988	
			Absolute	Percent
All causes				
Men	35–54	501	−189	−37.6
	55–74	2817	−646	−22.9
	75–84	9442	−1691	−17.9
	≥ 85	18549	213[a]	+1.1
Women	35–54	264	−72	−27.1
	55–74	1378	−237	−17.2
	75–84	5992	−1529	−25.5
	≥ 85	15115	−686	−4.5
Total cardiovascular disease deaths				
Men	35–54	224	−109	−48.5
	55–74	1626	−634	−39.0
	75–84	6002	−2080	−34.7
	≥ 85	12742	−2607	−20.5
Women	35–54	65	−26	−40.2
	55–74	679	−270	−39.7
	75–84	4083	−1730	−42.4
	≥ 85	11210	−2435	−21.7
Total cancer deaths				
Men	35–54	95	−16	−16.9
	55–74	615	+58	+9.4
	75–84	1582	+160	+10.2
	≥ 85	2051	+488	+23.8
Women	35–54	104	−9	−2.2
	55–74	423	+31	+14.0
	75–84	923	+42[a]	+8.1
	≥ 85	1324	+94	+7.6
Total noncardiovascular, noncancer deaths				
Men	35–54	182	−64	−35.1
	55–74	576	−70	−12.2
	75–84	1859	+228	+12.2
	≥ 85	3756	+2332	+62.1
Women	35–54	94	−35	−37.8
	55–74	277	0[a]	+0.1
	75–84	986	+160	+16.2
	≥ 85	2581	+1654	+64.1

[a] Not statistically significant; all others are statistically significant.

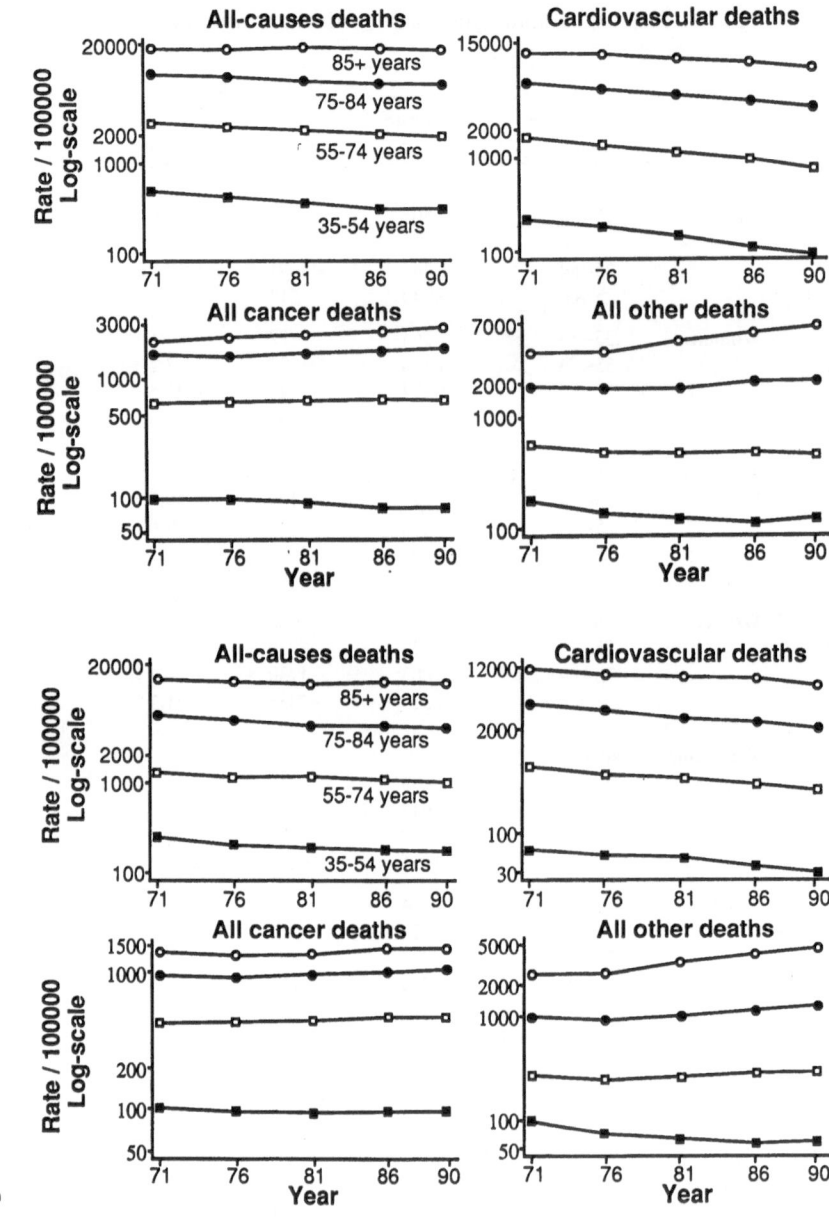

Fig. 1. Time trends of all causes, cardiovascular, cancer, and noncancer and non-cardiovascular mortality rates per 100 000, in Minnesota, according to age group, plotted on the logarithmic scale. Mortality rates are averaged for 1969–1973, 1974–1978, 1979–1983, 1984–1988, and 1989–1991 (plotted at years 1971, 1976, 1981, 1986, and 1990, respectively). Note that vertical scales differ between men and women, **a** men (*upper*), **b** women (*lower*)

Table 2. Trends in specific causes of death in Minnesota, 1969–1991, based on death-certificate ICD codes (underlying cause).

Death rates decreasing	Death rates steady	Death rates increasing
Coronary heart disease	Upper gastrointestinal,	Arrhythmias/congestive heart failure
Arterial embolism and	pancreatic, bladder and	Aortic aneurysm (men ≥ 75 years old)
thrombosis	kidney, breast, and	Natural causes
Hemorrhagic stroke	ovarian cancers	Ill-defined sudden death
Subarachnoid hemorrhage		Lung, liver, brain, and prostate
(< 75 years old)		cancers
Other stroke		Lymphatic/hematopoietic cancer (≥
Colorectal, stomach,		85 years old)
uterine, and cervical		Chronic obstructive pulmonary disease
cancers		Digestive system (≥ 85 years old)
Accidents and adverse		Endocrine and metabolic disease,
effects		except diabetes
Pneumonia (< 85 years		AIDS (men < 55 years old)
old)		Septicemia (≥ 55 years old)
Digestive system, including		Senility without psychosis (≥ 75 years
liver cirrhosis (< 85		old)
years old)		Senile dementia (≥ 75 years old)
Diabetes mellitus (< 85		Residual causes of death (> age 75)
years old)		

ICD codes, codes from World Health Organization, *International Classification of Diseases*.
Increase or decrease is judged to occur, depending on statistical significance of the absolute change in average annual death rate for 1984–1988 versus 1969–1973. See text for more details about extent of change in the rates of the causes of death listed above.

in total CVD death rates. However, the rate of decline in nonhemorrhagic stroke slowed after 1983, and the rate of hemorrhagic stroke death increased slightly between 1984–1988 and again between 1989–1991. Diabetes death rates decreased by about 20% in people below age 84, but were stable in those over age 85. Rates of several other causes of death decreased between 1969–1973 and 1984–1988: colorectal cancer (decreased about 15%, rates stable above age 85), stomach cancer (decreased about 40%), uterine and cervical cancers (each decreased about 40%; rates of ovarian cancer were stable), trauma (decreased about 40% below age 85 and 20% above age 85; suicide and homicide were stable), pneumonia and influenza (decreased about 25%, stable above age 85), and digestive diseases (decreased about 20% in men and 10% in women below age 84, but increased 30% in both genders above age 85).

Some cardiovascular diseases increased in frequency, including causes likely to represent more advanced forms of coronary heart disease, such as death attributed to arrhythmias and congestive heart failure (rates of which increased by as much as fivefold for ages greater than 55); aortic aneurysms in men age 75 or over (increased about 50%); and "natural causes" (increased by as much as sixfold above age 55). Death rates attributed to several forms of cancer showed upward trends. Lung cancer rates decreased by 20% in men aged 35–54, but increased by 28% to 116% in men over age 55 and increased by as much as threefold in women in all four age groups. Rates of liver and brain cancer death doubled at all ages; rates of prostate cancer increased by 20% at all ages. Rates of death attributed to lymphatic/hematopoietic cancer increased by 40% in people over age 85.

Rates of death attributed to chronic obstructive pulmonary disease doubled in men and tripled in women over age 55. Rates of endocrine and metabolic causes of death, other than diabetes, increased, more than doubling above age 85. AIDS death rates increased in younger men. Rates of death due to septicemia increased by threefold to eightfold in men and women over age 55. Death due to senility without psychosis doubled above age 85. Death due to senile dementia was rare before 1978, and increased 10- to 20-fold after 1979 in people over the age of 75. All residual death rates increased in older ages.

Levels and Change in Cardiovascular Risk Factors

Blood Pressure

Baseline blood pressure and prevalence of hypertension were greater in men than in women (Table 3a, Fig. 2). There was a tendency for systolic blood pressure (SBP) to decline in both sexes, greater in men over age 55 than in younger men, but not varying with age in women. Observed declines in diastolic blood pressure (DBP) were much shallower and more variable; they were not statistically significant in women. The DBP decline did not vary with age in men or women. There was a decline in the prevalence of hypertension, reflecting blood pressure decline throughout the blood pressure range. This did not vary with age in men, but was greater in women over age 44 ($>-1\%$ per year) than in women ages 25–44 (-0.27% per year).

Among hypertensives, prevalence of treatment to lower blood pressure was less in men than in women. Prevalence of unawareness of hypertension was (compensatorily) higher in men than in women. There was little variation in prevalence of treatment, or unawareness, over time or by age.

Body Mass Index

Body mass index (BMI) was greater in men than in women (Table 3b, Fig. 2). BMI increased steadily throughout the 1980s in both genders, at nearly twice the slope in women as in men. The change did not vary with age in men or women. Average height increased by about 0.3 cm during the decade, more so in men than in women.

Overweight, defined as BMI $\geq 27.5 \, \text{kg/m}^2$, was more prevalent in men than in women, and increased, with similar slopes in both genders, independent of age.

Table 3. Beseline levels and linear slopes for cardiovascular risk factors, Minnesota Heart Health Program, 1981–1990.

	Baseline, average 1981–1984		Change per year 1981–1990		P-value for slope
	Mean	SE	Slope	SE	different from 0
a. Blood pressure					
Systolic (mmHg)					
Men	124.7	0.24	−0.56[a]	0.07	0.0001
Women	116.4	0.46	−0.41	0.06	0.0001
P-value for sex difference	0.0001		0.1038		
Diastolic (mmHg)					
Men	77.7	0.2	−0.3	0.08	0.0003
Women	72.4	0.29	−0.09	0.07	0.1986
P-value for sex difference	0.0001		0.0483		
Hypertension (SBP/DBP ≥ 140/90 mmHg, or receiving medication) (%)					
Men	21.0	0.28	−0.58	0.17	0.0007
Women	13.6	0.38	−0.38	0.13	0.0036
P-value for sex difference	0.0001		0.3501		
Treatment to lower blood pressure (% among hypertensives)					
Men	39.9	0.16	0.65	0.4	0.1043
Women	56.5	0.11	0.36	0.36	0.3174
P-value for sex difference	0.0001		0.5901		
Unawareness of hypertension (% among hypertensives)					
Men	39.7	0.11	−0.32	0.37	0.3872
Women	29.8	0.11	−0.37	0.33	0.2623
P-value for sex difference	0.0001		0.9198		
b. Body mass index					
Body mass index (kg/m^2)					
Men	26.5	0.13	0.06	0.016	0.0003
Women	25.1	0.18	0.11	0.019	0.0001
P-value for sex difference	0.0001		0.0442		
Overweight (BMI ≥ 27.5 kg/m^2) (%)					
Men	33.2	0.14	0.67	0.2	0.0009
Women	23.7	0.15	0.69	0.15	0.0001
P-value for sex difference	0.0001		0.9363		
Caloric intake (Kcal/day)					
Men	2411.6	0.20	−19.69	5.64	0.0006
Women	1588.0	0.18	−0.23	3.46	0.9474
P-value for sex difference	0.0001		0.8185		
c. Cigarette smoking					
Current smoker (%)					
Men	34.4	0.17	−1.17	0.18	0.0001
Women	30.6	0.15	−0.67	0.17	0.0002
P-value for sex difference	0.0001		0.0435		

Table 3. *Continued.*

	Baseline, average 1981–1984		Change per year 1981–1990		P-value for slope different from 0
	Mean	SE	Slope	SE	
d. Serum cholesterol					
Serum cholesterol (mg/dl)					
Men	208.2	0.23	−1.02	0.23	0.0001
Women	203.7	0.44	−0.95	0.20	0.0001
P-value for sex difference	0.0001		0.8185		
Elevated serum cholesterol (serum cholesterol > 240) (%)					
Men	18.2	0.17	−0.62	0.18	0.0007
Women	13.1	0.31	−0.47	0.12	0.0002
P-value for sex difference	0.0001		0.4882		
Treatment to lower serum cholesterol (%)					
Men	0.19	0.09	0.16	0.04	0.0002
Women	0.05	0.08	0.13	0.03	0.0001
P-value for sex difference	0.2451		0.5486		
Keys score (mg/dl) (estimated)					
Men	47.2	0.09	−0.74	0.07	0.0001
Women	45.4	0.10	−0.87	0.08	0.0001
P-value for sex difference	0.0001		0.8185		
e. Physical activity					
Regular physical activity in leisure time (%)					
Men	52.1	0.15	0.72	0.21	0.0007
Women	46.3	0.17	1.16	0.20	0.0001
P-value for sex difference	0.0001		0.1293		
Total leisure time physical activity (Kcal/day)					
Men	291	0.14	−1.90	1.68	0.2582
Women	168	0.15	−0.99	0.85	0.2442
P-value for sex difference	0.0001		0.6290		
Heavy-intensity leisure time physical activity (Kcal/day)					
Men	91	0.18	−0.19	0.96	0.8432
Women	28	0.19	0.71	0.32	0.0266
P-value for sex difference	0.0001		0.3739		
Moderate-intensity leisure time physical activity (Kcal/day)					
Men	93	0.10	−1.53	0.56	0.0064
Women	70	0.13	−2.20	0.44	0.0001
P-value for sex difference	0.0001		0.3469		
Light-intensity leisure time physical activity (Kcal/day)					
Men	87	0.11	−1.17	0.58	0.0438
Women	59	0.14	0.43	0.42	0.3060
P-value for sex difference	0.0001		0.0256		

[a] Minus sign indicates decline.

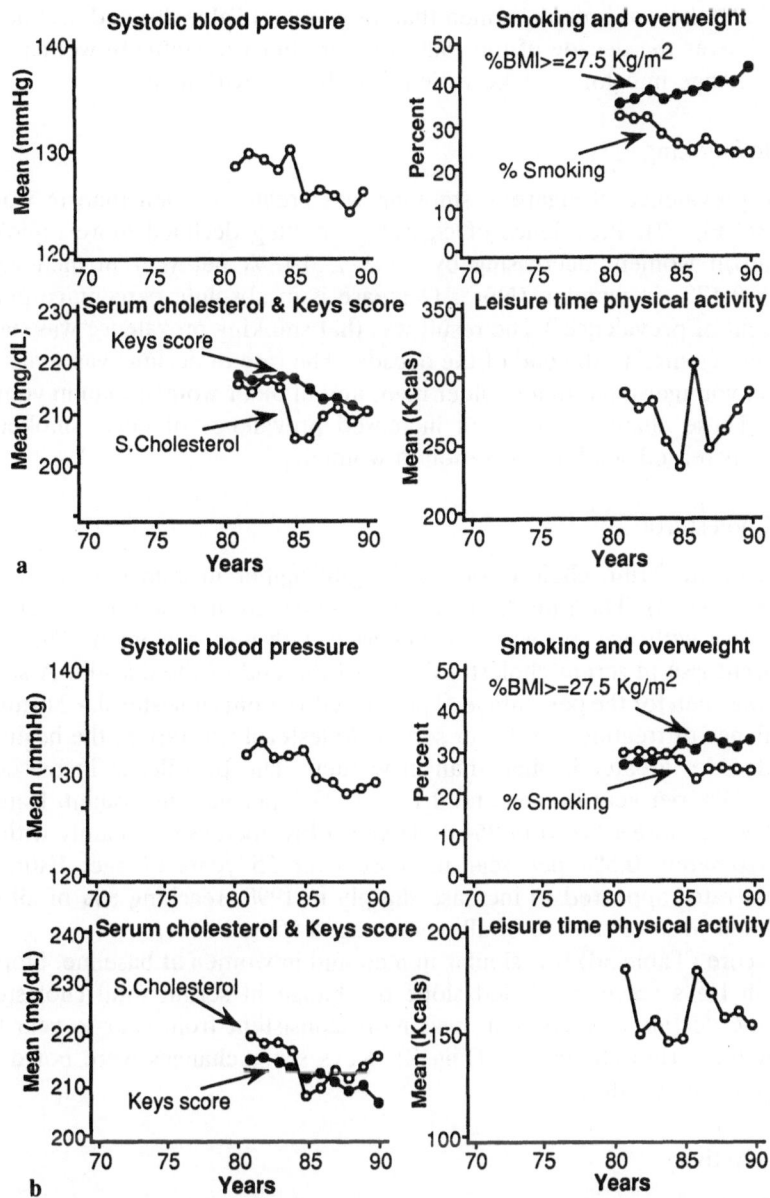

Fig. 2. Risk-factor trends based on Minnesota Heart Health Program serial cross-sectional surveys carried out between 1981 and 1990 of six communities in Minnesota, North Dakota, and South Dakota. The same calendar-year scale is used as in Fig. 1 to emphasize that risk-factor information is available in this study only during the latter half of the period of mortality observation, **a** men (*upper*), **b** women (*lower*)

Caloric intake was greater in men than in women (Table 3b) and declined by about 8% over the decade of the 1980s in men, but was stable in women. The slope of change in caloric intake varied little by age within gender.

Cigarette Smoking

Baseline prevalence of cigarette smoking was greater in men than in women (Table 3c, Fig. 2). Prevalence of cigarette smoking declined more rapidly in men than in women, decreasing by $-1.2 \pm 0.18\%$ per year in men versus $-0.67 \pm 0.17\%$ in women. (Note: Decrease is in absolute percentage points, not percent of prevalence.) The result was that smoking prevalence was similar in men and women at the end of the decade. The rate of decline was somewhat greater in younger men than in older men, and in older women than in younger women. These changes reflect an increased prevalence of never-smokers in men and increased smoking cessation in women.

Serum Cholesterol

Baseline mean serum cholesterol was 5 mg/dl higher in men than in women (Table 3d, Fig. 2). The rate of decline was similar in men and in women, and did not vary with age in men, but increased with age in women. There was an apparent rise in serum cholesterol toward the end of the decade. A similar pattern was seen for the percentage of people with serum cholesterol> 240 mg/dl.

Prevalence of treatment to lower serum cholesterol was rare at the beginning of the decade, greater in men than in women. The prevalence increased by $0.16 \pm 0.04\%$ per year in men and $0.13 \pm 0.03\%$ per year in women. Rates of increase were close to zero in 25- to 44-year-olds, increasing steadily with age to approximately 0.5% per year in those over 55 years of age. Estimated treatment rates appeared to increase sharply in 1990, reaching 8% of all men aged 45 and over versus 4% of all women aged 55 and over.

Keys score (Table 3d) was similar in men and in women at baseline. Slope of change in Keys score paralleled slope of change in serum total cholesterol, though the decline in Keys score was more consistent from year to year than was that for serum cholesterol (Fig. 2). Keys score changes were not differential by age or gender.

Physical Activity

Physical activity was measured in two ways, with a single question concerning prevalence of regular physical activity in leisure time, and with an extensive questionnaire in a random half of the subjects. Prevalence of reported regular physical activity in leisure time (Table 3e), as well as caloric expenditure per day, was greater in men than in women. Prevalence of regular physical activity in leisure time, assessed with the single question, increased in both men and women, the rate of increase being greater in people aged ≥ 45 than in people aged 25–44 years.

Results were different for time trends using the extensive Minnesota Leisure Time Physical Activity Questionnaire. Caloric expenditure (Table 3e, Fig. 2) declined by −10 Kcal/day per year in men aged 25–44, did not change in men aged 45–64, and increased by 9 Kcal/day per year in men aged 65–74. Caloric expenditure in leisure time physical activity did not change in any age group in women. Caloric expenditure in heavy-intensity leisure time physical activities decreased in men aged 25–44, and did not change in older men. It increased in women, independent of age. Caloric expenditure in moderate-intensity leisure time physical activities decreased in men aged 25–44 and increased in men aged 65–74 years. It decreased in women, independent of age. Caloric expenditure in light-intensity leisure time physical activities decreased in men aged 25–44, and did not change in older men. It did not change in women, independent of age.

Discussion

In recent decades, Minnesota has experienced major declines in mortality rates, driven largely by declines in coronary heart disease and stroke deaths. Large declines in CVD deaths were complemented by declines in rates of other major categories of death at ages 35–54, but were slightly offset by increases in cancer death rates at ages 55–74. About 10–20% of the decline in total CVD deaths observed at age 75–84 was "compensated" by increases in cancer and other causes of death. Even at ages ≥ 85, the oldest age-at-death category in the Minnesota Department of Health death certificate data base, the increase in noncardiovascular death rates just matched the decrease in CVD deaths. Therefore, death rates in the oldest age group were stable, despite the delay in death rates implied by the reduced rates at younger ages. Rates for several causes of death increased, mostly in people over age 75 or 85. However, death rates increased substantially at ages above 55 in several common conditions, including arrhythmias and congestive heart failure; lung, brain, liver, and prostate cancers; chronic obstructive pulmonary disease; endocrine and metabolic conditions (excluding diabetes mellitus); and septicemia.

Risk-factor trends were generally favorable (from the perspective of reducing CHD risk), with the exception of a trend to increasing body mass index. Changes in physical activity were equivocal, showing increases when measured with a simple questionnaire, but decreases when measured with a more detailed one. We have no explanation for the difference in physical activity outcome according to the measurement strategy. The decline in caloric intake by men suggests decreased physical activity. These risk-factor changes, occurring during the last decade covered by the mortality analysis, continued the pattern of earlier years [3–10].

We suppose that the decline in atherosclerotic coronary heart disease and stroke death rates was mediated in part by risk-factor changes, particularly reductions in smoking, blood cholesterol and blood pressure. The reduction

in cigarette smoking was greater in men than women. Change in blood cholesterol closely paralleled changes in Keys score, and therefore appeared to be
mediated by dietary change. The prevalence of drug treatment to lower blood
cholesterol is still low, though it has risen sharply in recent years. Change in
blood pressure has likely been influenced by use of medication, but decreases
in blood pressure have occurred throughout the entire distribution: Medication
alone, therefore, cannot explain entirely the fall in population-wide levels of
blood pressure [13].

Two aspects of analysis of underlying causes from death certificates are
problematic. The ICD code change in 1979 from ICD-8 to ICD-9 may artifi-
cially change the rate of a given cause of death. We have considered published
comparability ratios between ICD-8 and ICD-9 coding [14], and do not believe
that the change in coding systems explains much of the change in death rates
found in this study, because the comparability ratios are generally small compared to the observed changes in mortality rates. A potentially more serious
problem is ignoring contributing causes listed on the death certificate. Coronary
heart disease is recognized as the underlying cause in most cases in which it is
listed on the death certificate; but it is unclear what is missed by not recog-
nizing the presence of diseases such as septicemia, which is rarely coded as the
underlying cause of death. Nevertheless, the increase in selected causes of
death in middle age is worthy of further investigation.

We note several candidate explanations for the increase in rates of several
causes of death:

1. Both cancer and noncancer lung disease develop over decades and are
strongly influenced by cigarette smoking. It is likely that current rates of these
diseases reflect the smoking habits over the past 20 or more years. The pattern
of change in rate of lung cancer death fits this explanation, in that the youngest
men (aged 35–54) showed a decline in rates; older men showed an increase in
rates, but at a slower rate than women aged 35–84; and women over age 85
(relatively few of whom ever smoked) showed a less steep increase than
younger women.

2. In many diseases, increasing death rates are restricted to ages over 75 or
85. Increasing death rates may therefore reflect general deterioration in older
people who did not succumb from atherosclerosis.

3. Several manifestations of CHD, such as arrhythmias and congestive heart
failure, may have increased as a result of successful ameliorative treatment of
CHD and stroke.

4. Some changes are the result of changes in diagnostic fashion, for example,
the increased use of the rubric "natural causes" by physicians and pathologists
in this region.

5. There may be deleterious effects from certain risk-factor changes, as
considered in a recent conference [15,16], and vigorously disputed by others
[17] for low (or lowered) levels of blood cholesterol. Such an effect might occur
in causes of death where rates are increasing, in which secondary effects

from successful treatment of coronary heart disease or stroke are an unlikely explanation.

In conclusion, risk-factor reduction that has occurred in Minnesota for the past several decades seems to be highly beneficial in reduction of most causes of death. Nevertheless, increases in rates of selected causes of death appear worthy of ongoing attention, and continued surveillance of mortality, morbidity, and risk factors is therefore advisable to detect unexpected occurrences.

Acknowledgements. Supported by NIH Grants R01-HL-23727 (Minnesota Heart Survey) and R01-HL-25523 (Minnesota Heart Health Program).

References

1. Goldman L, Cook EF (1984) The decline in ischemic heart disease mortality rates. An analysis of the comparative effects of medical interventions and changes in lifestyle. Ann Intern Med 101:825–1836.
2. Gilbertson DT, McGovern PG, Jacobs DR, Gatewood LG, Blackburn H (1992) A mathematical modeling approach toward explaining the decline in coronary heart disease mortality. Circulation 86, abstract no 2378
3. Department of Health and Human Services (1972) Blood pressure levels in persons 18–74 years of age in 1976–1980, and trends in blood pressure from 1960 to 1980 in the United States. National Center for Health Statistics, Hyattsville, Md. (Series II: Data from the National Health Survey, no 234) (DHHS publication no (PHS) 86-1684)
4. National Center for Health Statistics, National Heart, Lung and Blood Institute Collaboration Lipid Group (1987) Trends in serum cholesterol levels among US adults aged 20 to 74 years. Data from the National Health and Nutrition Examination Surveys, 1960 to 1980. JAMA 257:937–942
5. Johnson CL, Rifkind BM, Sempos CT, Carroll MD, Bachorik PS, Briefel RR, Gordon DJ, Burt VL, Brown CD, Lippel K, Cleeman JI (1993) Declining serum total cholesterol levels among US adults. The National Health and Nutrition Examination Surveys. JAMA 269:3002–3008
6. Fiore ML, Novotny TE, Pierce JP, Hatziandreu EJ, Patel KM, Davies RM (1989) Trends in cigarette smoking in the United States. The changing influence of gender and race. JAMA 261:49–55
7. Jacobs D (1978) Risk factor changes in Minneapolis men. In: Proceedings of the Conference on the Decline in Coronary Heart Disease Mortality. U.S. Department of Health, Education and Welfare, Bethesda, Md. NIH publication no 79–1610, pp 215–217
8. Sprafka JM, Burke GL, Folsom AR, Luepker RV, Blackburn H (1990) Continued decline in cardiovascular disease risk factors: Results of the Minnesota Heart Survey, 1980–1982 and 1985–1987. Am J Epidemiol 132:489–500
9. Luepker RV, Jacobs DR, Folsom AR, Gillum RF, Frantz ID, Gomez-Marin O, Blackburn H (1988) Cardiovascular risk factor change 1973–74 to 1980–82: The Minnesota Heart Survey. J Clin Epidemiol 41:825–833

10. Jacobs DR, Hahn LP, Folsom AR, Hannan PJ, Sprafka JM, Burke GL (1991) Time trends in leisure-time physical activity in the Upper Midwest 1957–1987: University of Minnesota Studies. Epidemiology 2:8–15
11. Jacobs DR Jr, Luepker RV, Mittelmark MB, Folsom AR, Pirie PL, Mascioli SR, Hannan PJ, Pechacek TF, Bracht NF, Carlaw RW, Kline FG, Blackburn H, for the Minnesota Heart Health Program Research Group (1986) Community-wide prevention strategies: Evaluation design of the Minnesota Heart Health Program. J Chronic Dis 39:775–788
12. Mittelmark MB, Luepker RV, Jacobs DR, Bracht NF, Carlaw RW, Crow RS, Finnegan J, Grimm RH, Jeffery RW, Kline FG, Mullis RM, Murray DM, Pechacek TF, Perry CL, Pirie PL, Blackburn H, for the Minnesota Heart Health Program Research Group (1986) Community-wide prevention of cardiovascular disease: Education strategies of the Minnesota Heart Health Program. Prev Med 15:1–17
13. Jacobs DR, McGovern PG, Blackburn H (1992) Why is stroke mortality declining? Is ecologic analysis informative? Am J Publ Health 82:1596–1599
14. Klebba AJ, Scott JH (1980) Estimates of selected comparability ratios based on dual coding of 1976 death certificates by the eighth and ninth revisions of the International Classification of Diseases. Monthly Vital Statistics Report. Department of Health Education and Welfare publication no PHS 80-1120, vol 28, no 11[Suppl]
15. Jacobs D, Blackburn H, Higgins M, Reed D, Iso H, McMillan G, Neaton J, Nelson J, Potter J, Rifkind B, Rossouw J, Shekelle R, Yusuf S (1992) Report of the Conference on Low Blood Cholesterol: Mortality Associations. Circulation 86:1046–1060
16. Jacobs DR (1993) Why is low blood cholesterol associated with risk of nonatherosclerotic disease death? Ann Rev Publ Health 14:95–114
17. Stamler J, Stamler R, Brown WV, Gotto AM, Greenland P, Grundy S, Hegsted DM, Luepker RV, Neaton JD, Steinberg D, Stone N, Van Horn L, Wissler RW (1993) Serum cholesterol. Doing the right thing. Circulation 88:1954–1960

Discussion

A. Dontas: You have commented on the mortality in the U.S. Midwest since about 1969. I have the impression that risk factor changes occurred there earlier. Would you comment on this lag between risk factor and mortality change?

D. Jacobs: I have little information about what happened to risk factors in the U.S. before our Minnesota population-based surveys starting in the early 1970s. I mentioned the LRC survey conducted by Henry Taylor that suggested changes from 1966–75. This is confirmed by Framingham Study findings that risk factors were higher in the 1950s and 1960s, but I can't give a definitive answer on that interesting question.

M. Karvonen: One gets rather unusual results from using open-ended age groups. Age groups open above 20 or 50 or 85 years may give quite unusual results.

D. Jacobs: You are justifiably critical of the selection of age 85. We have also done the analysis with age 75+ as cut-off. I was a little surprised to see also substantial mortality declines in the 75–85 age group. Perhaps if I broke out age 85 and beyond into separate, smaller age groups, I would continue to be surprised. Good point.

R. Beaglehole: Dr. Jacobs, I was impressed with the variety of analyses presented in these last papers and the degree of enthusiasm with which some of the presenters were able to relate the trends in risk factors to the trends in mortality. You, on the other hand, were particularly cautious in your summing up, and I wonder if you would like to make some comments about the methods we are currently using to look at these parallel trends in risk factors and mortality.

D. Jacobs: I have no specific concern about the variety of methods used epidemiologically. The caution I expressed is only because I believe we can feel confident with the general pattern of risk factor reduction that appears to have occurred in some populations and cultures, and because this decline seems to have had a beneficial effect in many areas of mortality and health.

This does not mean, however, that every component of different risk factor patterns is optimal, especially here in Japan where we may be seeing the beginning of an increase in CHD incidence, and where there has been in the past such a large burden of hemorrhagic stroke, which is now clearly diminished. All this indicates we must continue careful research on these issues. I am cautious because of the rapid changes happening in Japan, a culture very much in transition.

Socioeconomic Differences in Trends in Coronary Heart Disease Mortality and Risk Factors in Finland

Juha Pekkanen, Antti Uutela, Tapani Valkonen,
Erkki Vartiainen, Jaakko Tuomilehto, and Pekka Puska

Summary. Finland has witnessed a rapid decline in coronary heart disease (CHD) mortality among working-age men and women since the end of the 1960s. Among men aged 35–64, age-standardized CHD mortality declined by 50% from 1971–1972 to 1990–1991. The trend has been similar among women. Concomitant with the declining mortality, there have been improvements in the levels of CHD risk factors. In the provinces of North Karelia and Kuopio, risk-factor surveys have been carried out among independent random samples of the middle-aged population every 5 years since 1972. In these surveys, improvements have been observed in mean serum total cholesterol concentration, diastolic blood pressure, and smoking. Although overall changes have been favorable, relative differences in CHD mortality between educational groups have widened, especially in the 1980s in Finland. In risk factors, the decline in serum cholesterol and in the proportion of hypertensives among both sexes, and in smoking among men, has been similar in all educational groups. However, trends in body mass index have diverged between educational groups, and among women, smoking has changed from a habit of the more educated to a habit of the less educated.

Key words. Coronary heart disease—Mortality—Risk factors—Education—Time trends

Introduction

Coronary heart disease (CHD) mortality has declined among the middle-aged population in most, though not all, industrial countries [1]. Finland experienced a rapid decline in CHD mortality among working-age men and women after the end of the 1960s [2].

Although overall changes in CHD mortality have been favorable, relative differences in mortality between socioeconomic groups have grown during the 1980s in Finland [3,4]. There is evidence for similar development in England during the 1970s [5], and in the United States [6,7].

In Finland [8,9], as in most other industrial countries [10], lower socioeconomic groups tend to have a more adverse cardiovascular risk-factor profile. There are also a few reports suggesting growing socioeconomic differences in the prevalence of cardiovascular risk factors, especially in smoking [11–16].

The aim of this chapter is first to describe overall trends in CHD mortality among the middle-aged population in Finland and the concomitant changes in cardiovascular risk factors in eastern Finland. Secondly, CHD mortality and risk-factor trends by education are presented.

Methods

Mortality Data

The mortality data for the years 1951–1991 (Fig. 1) have been derived from published statistics of Statistics Finland [2]. The data on mortality by level of education (Fig. 2) are based on the death records for the years 1971–1991, which have been linked with the individual level records of the censuses carried out in Finland in 1970, 1975, 1980, and in 1985 [3,4]. The computerized linkage of records was carried out by Statistics Finland by means of personal identification numbers used in Finland. The data cover all deaths from coronary heart disease (World Health Organization, *International Classification of Diseases*, code 410–414) in the age group 35–64 from 1971–1991 (55 100 male and 10 300 female deaths). The 3-year averages of death rates presented in Fig. 2 are, as a rule, based on several hundreds of deaths. The only exceptions are the death rates for women with 13 or more years of education, which are based on 100–200 deaths. The age-standardized death rates were calculated by the direct method using the 1966–1970 stationary population as the standard population.

Risk-Factor Data

Cross-sectional population surveys in 1972, 1977, 1982, and 1987 assessed the levels of coronary risk factors in the provinces of North Karelia and Kuopio in 5-year intervals. In North Karelia, an intensive community-wide multifactorial cardiovascular disease prevention program was started in 1972 [17]. For each survey, an independent random sample was drawn from the national population register. In the 1972 and 1977 surveys, a random sample of 6.6% of the population born during 1913–1947 was drawn in both areas. In 1982 and 1987, the sample included persons aged 25–64 years. The samples were stratified so that at least 250 subjects of each sex and 10-year age group were chosen in each area. The common age range in all of the surveys was 30–59 years, which is the age range of risk-factor data used in the present analyses.

The survey methods followed the World Health Organization (WHO) MONICA protocol in 1982 and 1987 [18] and they were comparable with the methods used in 1972 and 1977. The surveys included a self-administered

Fig. 1. Age-standardized coronary heart disease mortality (per 100 000 population) in 1951–1991 among men and women aged 35–64 in Finland

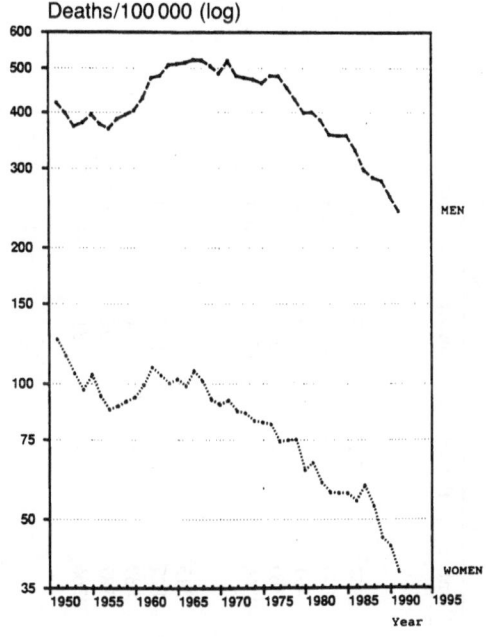

Fig. 2. Age-standardized coronary heart disease mortality (per 100 000 population) in 1971–1991 by years of education among men and women aged 35–64, in Finland. Three-year moving averages

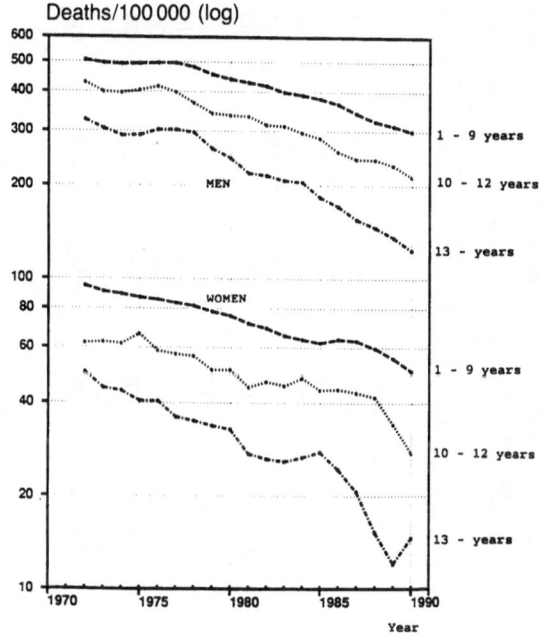

Table 1. Number of those examined by education. Men and women aged 30–59 in Eastern Finland.

	1972		1977		1982		1987	
	Number	Percent	Number	Percent	Number	Percent	Number	Percent
Men								
Years of education								
≤7	2401	55	1903	44	857	36	445	36
8	1049	24	1191	28	649	27	455	26
9–11	561	13	712	16	491	21	480	28
≥12	395	9	549	13	369	16	351	21
All	4406	100	4355	100	2366	100	1731	100
Level of education[a]								
Low	835	19	837	19	513	22	392	23
Medium	1507	34	1544	36	827	35	519	30
Higher	1320	30	1238	28	639	27	514	30
Highest	726	17	736	17	387	16	306	18
All	4406	100	4355	100	2366	100	1731	100
Women								
Years of education								
≤7	2385	51	1777	39	609	28	375	20
8	1028	22	1168	26	563	26	388	21
9–11	813	18	1034	23	571	26	619	34
≥12	433	9	573	13	445	20	457	25
All	4659	100	4552	100	2188	100	1839	100
Level of education[a]								
Low	685	15	662	15	320	15	323	17
Medium	1452	31	1368	30	617	28	439	24
Higher	1594	34	1659	36	780	36	693	38
Highest	928	20	863	19	471	21	384	21
All	4659	100	4552	100	2188	100	1839	100

[a] Level of education relative to each person's 5-year birth cohort.

questionnaire, blood sampling, and measurements of height, weight, and blood pressure. Methods have been presented in detail elsewhere [17–19].

Smoking was assessed in all surveys using exactly the same questionnaire. Serum cholesterol was determined, from frozen samples using the Liebermann–Burchard method in 1972 and 1977, whereas in 1982 and 1987, serum cholesterol was determined from fresh sera using an enzymatic method (CHOD-PAP, Boehringer Mannheim, Germany, Monotest). The enzymatic assay method gave 2.4% lower values than the Liebermann–Burchard method. Cholesterol values of the 1972 and 1977 surveys were corrected for this bias in Table 2. In 1972 and 1977, blood pressures were measured with a shorter cuff bladder (23 cm) than in 1982 and in 1987 (42 cm). Also the survey question on antihypertensive medication changed slightly in 1982. Participation rates were very high, more than 90%, in both areas and both sexes in the first survey in 1972. The proportion participating decreased slightly over time, but remained satisfactory. The lowest participation rate, 77%, was observed among men in North Karelia in 1982.

In the analysis, current smokers and smokers who had quit smoking during the last half year were classified as smokers. Hypertension was defined as systolic blood pressure over 159 mmHg, diastolic blood pressure over 94 mmHg, or use of antihypertensive medication.

Years of education was always asked with the same question: "How many years have you had school altogether or studied full-time in your life?" The average level of education has increased significantly during the past 20 years in Finland. Therefore, in order to obtain equal-sized groups for different study years, each 5-year birth cohort, men and women included, was divided into four educational categories. For each cohort, the mode year for the years of education was determined and named the "medium" group. Those with less education than the mode were called the "low" group. About 20% of the subjects with the most education were termed the "highest" group. The remaining subjects belonged to the "higher" group. Results were, however, analyzed also using the absolute cut-points shown in Table 1. The conclusions from these analyses were identical to those presented.

Educational differences in risk factors were analyzed using logistic regression models for categorical variables and analysis of covariance for continuous variables. No trend tests were used; education was always treated as a categorical variable with three degrees of freedom ($df = 3$). All models used included year of examination, living area, and age. Socioeconomic differences in risk-factor trends were tested by entering into the model an interaction term between education and year of examination ($df = 9$).

Results

Among the middle-aged men in Finland, CHD mortality increased from the late 1950s and early 1960s and then declined starting in the early 1970s (Fig. 1). The decline was 50% from 1971/1972 to 1990/1991. Among women, the rapid

Table 2. Risk factor levels among men and women aged 30–59 in Eastern Finland.

	1972		1977		1982		1987	
	Mean	SD	Mean	SD	Mean	SD	Mean	SD
Men								
Cholesterol (mmol/l)	6.78	1.27	6.55	1.23	6.28	1.20	6.23	1.21
Diastolic blood pressure (mmHg)	92.8		91.0	11.7	87.8	13.0	88.4	11.6
Smoking (%)	53	12.0	47		42		39	
Women								
Cholesterol (mmol/l)	6.72	1.33	6.36	1.31	6.10	1.30	5.94	1.22
Diastolic blood pressure (mmHg)	91.8	12.7	87.6	11.5	84.6	11.9	83.5	11.4
Smoking (%)	11		12		16		16	

decline started at about the same time and was about equally fast compared with men, 54% from 1971/1972 to 1990/91.

Risk-factor surveys among independent random samples of the provinces of North Karelia and Kuopio Counties have been carried out every 5 years since 1972 (Table 1). In these surveys, mean serum total cholesterol decreased continuously from 1972 to 1987, both among men and among women (Table 2). Decreases were also observed in mean diastolic blood pressure. Changes appear to have been more rapid in the 1970s than in the 1980s. The prevalence of smoking among men decreased from 53% to 39%, but it increased among women from 11% to 16%.

Although CHD mortality has declined in all socioeconomic groups, the relative decline has been faster among the higher socioeconomic groups. Among men with 13 or more years of education, the decline in CHD mortality from 1971–1972 to 1990–1991 was 66%, among men with 10–12 years of education it was 54%, and among men with less than 10 years of education it was 43% (Fig. 2). Among women, the respective declines were 72%, 63%, and 46%. In the early 1970s the relative decline was similar in all educational groups, but after the late 1970s the trends started to diverge between the educational groups. The absolute differences between educational groups have, however, narrowed slightly.

The level of education increased rapidly after 1972, when the first surveys in North Karelia and Kuopio were carried out (Table 1). To be able to compare socioeconomic differences in trends of risk factors, a classification based on level of education relative to each person's 5-year birth cohort was used. Statistically significant educational differences in all risk factors examined were observed both among men and women. Among men, the only significant educational difference in trends was the divergence of the mean body mass index trend (interaction between year of examination and education $P < 0.001$) (Fig. 3). In 1972 the least-educated men tended to have the lowest mean body mass index. However, due to the rapid increase in body mass index in the

Fig. 3. Age-standardized cardio-vascular risk-factor levels by education among eastern Finnish men aged 30–59, 1972–1987

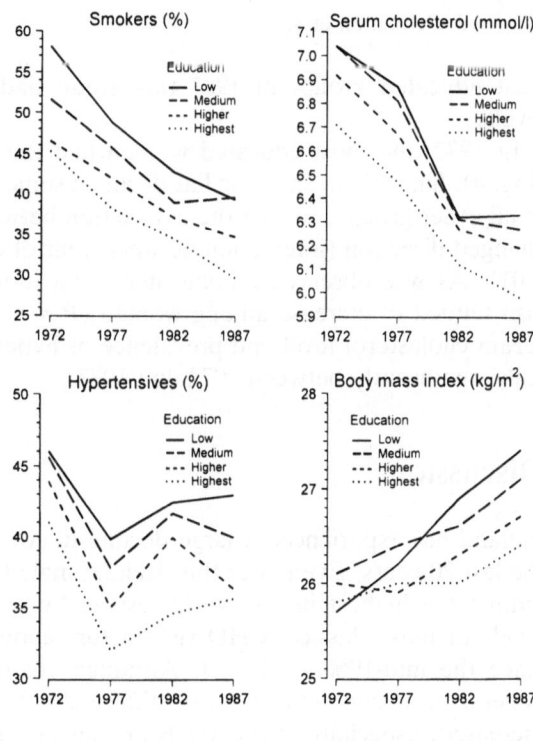

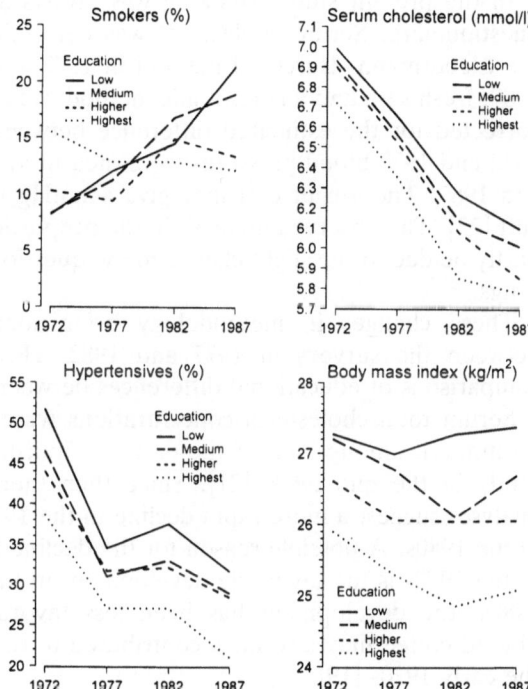

Fig. 4. Age-standardized cardio-vascular risk-factor levels by education among eastern Finnish women aged 30–59, 1972–1987

least educated group, in 1987 this group had the highest body mass index levels.

In 1972, the most educated women had the highest prevalence of smoking (Fig. 4). Since then, smoking has declined somewhat in this group but increased in all other groups, so that the association between education and smoking has changed direction (interaction between year of examination and education $P <$ 0.01). As was observed among men, educational differences in obesity have also tended to increase among women ($P = 0.06$). Educational differences in serum cholesterol level and prevalence of hypertension did not change statistically significantly between 1972 and 1987.

Discussion

Finland has experienced a large decline in coronary heart disease mortality in the last 20 years. Even after this decline, male CHD mortality in Finland is still among the highest in the world, especially in eastern Finland [20]. Average levels of most classical CHD risk factors appear to have declined in Finland since the mid-1960s [2,19,21]. Although changes in CHD mortality have in general been favorable, relative differences between educational groups have increased, especially in the 1980s in Finland. The present study also suggests that some increases in educational differences in risk-factor levels have taken place in eastern Finland.

In the present study, smoking was always assessed using exactly the same questionnaire. Serum cholesterol was determined from frozen samples using the Liebermann–Burchard method in 1972 and 1977, whereas in 1982 and in 1987, fresh sera and an enzymatic method were used. The means in Table 2 are corrected for the estimated difference between the methods, 2.4%. Also, in 1972 and 1977 blood pressures were measured with a shorter cuff than in 1982 and 1987. The longer cuff may give 4 mmHg lower readings than the shorter cuff [22]. The observed increase in the proportion of hypertensives in 1982 may partly be due to the slight change in the question on the use of antihypertensive drugs.

These changes in methodology bring some uncertainty in comparisons between the surveys in 1977 and 1982. However, they do not affect the comparisons of educational differences between surveys.

Serum total cholesterol concentrations were at their highest average level, 6.9 mmol/l, among men of the eastern Finnish cohort of the Seven Countries Study in the mid-1960s [21]. Since then there has been a decline. Present analyses suggest a more rapid decline in the 1970s and a slowing of the decline in the 1980s. A possible reason for the decline in mean serum cholesterol level in the 1970s is the favorable development in fat quality in Finland [19]. In the 1980s, the development has been less favorable. The shift from boiled to filtered coffee may also have contributed to the fall in serum cholesterol since the early 1970s [19].

Prevalence of smoking among men in Finland appears to have declined since the 1960s [2,21]. The decline slowed in the 1980s, and there has been an increase among women. In the 1970s, there was active discussion about forthcoming tobacco legislation, which may have contributed to the decline. After the late 1970s, no real improvements in smoking control occurred in Finland [19].

Although overall CHD mortality has declined, the present analyses show that relative differences between educational groups have increased, especially in the 1980s in Finland. The findings are similar when using occupation instead of education [3,4]. There is evidence for a similar development in England during the 1970s [5]. In the United States, educational differences in all-cause mortality appear to have increased between 1960 and 1986 [7]. Also, differences in CHD mortality between communities with differing occupational structure increased in the United States between 1968 and 1982 [6].

In Finland [8,9], as in most other industrial countries [10], lower socioeconomic groups tend to have a more adverse cardiovascular risk-factor profile. In addition, a significant part of the association between social class and coronary heart disease mortality is mediated through the known, preventable cardiovascular risk factors in Finland [9,23], as in many other industrial countries [24]. In a follow-up study of 8967 men and 9694 women aged 30–64 years, who were examined in 1972 and 1977 in connection with the North Karelia Project, lower social classes had higher mortality from all major causes [9]. Most CHD risk factors examined were also more common in the lower social classes. Among men, the age-adjusted relative risk for CHD death, comparing unskilled manual workers and upper-level nonmanual workers, was reduced from 1.55 (95% CI 1.17–2.04) to 1.23 (95% CI 0.93–1.62) when adjusting also for smoking, serum cholesterol, hypertension, body mass index, and leisure time physical activity. Among women, the corresponding reduction in relative risk was from 1.74 (95% CI 1.05–2.90) to 1.64 (95% CI 0.98–2.75).

There are a few reports suggesting growing socioeconomic differences in the prevalence of some cardiovascular risk factors. Two reports from the United States [11,12] and one from Sweden [13] showed growing socioeconomic differences in the prevalence of smoking, and a report from the United States suggested growing differences also in mean serum cholesterol level [14]. Reports on obesity have given mixed results [15,16].

In the present analyses, there was an increase in educational differences in body mass index among both sexes and in the prevalence of smoking among women. In mean serum cholesterol level and in the prevalence of hypertension, no change with time in educational differences was observed. The diverging trends in smoking may certainly have contributed to the diverging trends in CHD mortality among women. The significance of the diverging trends in mean body mass index is, in contrast, questionable. It is not clear whether body mass index is an independent risk factor for CHD when adjusting for smoking, serum cholesterol, and blood pressure [25]. It is also not clear which is cause and which is effect, low education or high body mass index [26]. Most probably the relation is bidirectional and may even be confounded by other factors, such as heredity [27]. High body mass index may partly reflect other factors that may have contributed to the diverging trends in CHD mortality.

Favorable changes in health behavior occur usually first in the higher social classes [28]. This may, at least temporarily, have increased relative mortality differences between the social classes. The experience from the North Karelia Project in the 1970s gave, however, indication that a community-wide intervention program may eventually have a favorable effect in every social group [29]. To decrease the health inequalities between social classes, present health promotion methods should be reevaluated and developed further to take into account especially the needs of the lower social classes. This by itself will probably not be sufficient, but increasing health inequalities need to be addressed at multiple levels, from general social policy to everyday practice [10].

A considerable part of the excess CHD mortality in lower social classes in Finland is mediated through the known, modifiable risk factors [9,23]. This suggests that it may be possible to narrow the social class differences in health through larger improvements in health behavior among the lower social classes. Trends in CHD mortality have been less favorable among the lower socioeconomic groups compared to higher socioeconomic groups [3,4]. There was also no evidence for diminishing socioeconomic differences in risk factors between educational groups in the present analyses, and even some evidence for increasing differences. This suggests that in the present analyses social inequalities in CHD mortality in Finland may well increase in the future if appropriate action is not taken.

References

1. Thom TJ (1989) International mortality from heart disease: rates and trends. Int Epidemiol 18[Suppl I]:S20–S28
2. Pyorala K, Salonen JT, Valkonen T (1985) Trends in coronary heart disease mortality and morbidity and related factors in Finland. Cardiology 72:35–51
3. Valkonen T, Martelin T, Rimpela A (1990) Socio-economic mortality differences in Finland 1971–85. Central Statistical Office of Finland, Studies 176, Helsinki
4. Valkonen T, Martelin T, Rimpela A, Notkola V, Savela S (1993) Socio-economic mortality differences in Finland 1981–90. Statistics Finland, Population 1, Helsinki
5. Marmot MG, McDowell ME (1986) Mortality decline and widening social inequalities. Lancet 2:274–276
6. Wing S, Dargent-Molina P, Casper M, Riggan W, Hayes CG, Tyroler HA (1987) Changing association between community occupational structure and ischemic heart disease mortality in the United States. Lancet 2:1067–1070
7. Pappas G, Queen S, Hadden W, Fisher G (1993) The increasing disparity in mortality between socioeconomic groups in the United States, 1960 and 1986. N Engl J Med 329:103–109

8. Tuomilehto J, Puska P, Virtamo J, Neittaanmaki L, Koskela K (1978) Coronary risk factors and socioeconomic status in Eastern Finland. Prev Med 7:539–549
9. Pekkanen J, Tuomilehto J, Uutela A, Vartiainen E, Nissinen A (1992) Social class, coronary risk factors, and mortality among eastern Finnish men and women (in Finnish). Duodecim 108:1395–1402
10. Adler NE, Boyce WT, Chesney MA, Folkman S, Syme SL (1993) Socioeconomic inequalities in health. No easy solution. JAMA 269:3140–3145
11. Pierce JP, Fiore MC, Novotny TE, Hatziandreu EJ, Davis RM (1989) Trends in cigarette smoking in the United States. JAMA 261:56–60
12. Covey LS, Zang EA, Wynder EL (1992) Cigarette smoking and occupational status: 1977 to 1990. Am J Publ Health 82:1230–1234
13. Rosen M, Hanning M, Wall S (1990) Changing smoking habits in Sweden: Towards better health, but not for all. Int J Epidemiol 19:316–322
14. National Center for Health Statistics (1987) Trends in serum cholesterol levels among US adults aged 20 to 74 years. JAMA 257:937–942
15. Flegal KM, Harlan WR, Landis JR (1988) Secular trends in body mass index and skinfold thickness with socioeconomic factors in young adult men. Am J Clin Nutr 48:544–551
16. Kuskowska-Wolk A, Bergstrom R (1993) Trends in body mass index and prevalence of obesity in Swedish men 1980–89. J Epidemiol Commun Health 47: 103–108
17. Puska P, Nissinen A, Tuomilehto J, Salonen JT, Koskela K, McAlister A, Kottke TE, Maccoby N, Farquhar JW (1985) The community-based strategy to prevent coronary heart disease: Conclusions from the ten years of the North Karelia Project. Ann Rev Publ Health 6:147–193
18. WHO MONICA Project (prepared by Tunstall-Pedoe H) (1988) The World Health Organization MONICA Project (monitoring trends and determinants in cardiovascular disease): major international collaboration. J Clin Epidemiol 41: 105–114
19. Vartiainen E, Korhonen HJ, Pietinen P, Tuomilehto J, Kartovaara L, Nissinen A, Puska P (1991) Fifteen-year trends in coronary risk factors in Finland, with special reference to North Karelia. Int J Epidemiol 20:651–662
20. WHO MONICA Project (prepared by Tuomilehto J, Kuulasmaa K, Torppa J) (1987) Geographic variation in mortality from cardiovascular diseases. Baseline data on selected population characteristics and cardiovascular mortality. World Health Stat Q 40:171–184
21. Pekkanen J (1987) Coronary heart disease during a 25–year follow-up. Risk factors and their secular trends in the Finnish cohorts of the Seven Countries Study. Academic dissertation. Health Services Research by the National Board of Health in Finland No. 45. Government Printing Centre, Helsinki
22. Nissinen A, Tuomilehto J, Korhonen HJ, Piha T, Salonen JT, Puska P (1988) Ten-year results of hypertension care in the community. Follow-up of the North Karelia hypertension control program. Am J Epidemiol 127:488–499
23. Salonen JT (1982) Socioeconomic status and risk of cancer, cerebral stroke, and death due to coronary heart disease and any disease: A longitudinal study in Eastern Finland. J Epidemiol Commun Health 36:294–297
24. Marmot MG, Shipley MJ, Rose G (1984) Inequalities in death-specific explanations of a general pattern? Lancet 1:1003–1006
25. Jarrett RJ (1986) Is there an ideal body weight? Br Med J 293:493–495

26. Gortmaker SL, Must A, Perrin JM, Sobol AM, Dietz WH (1993) Social and economic consequences of overweight in adolescence and young adulthood. N Engl J Med 329:1008–1012
27. Stunkard AJ, Sorensen TIA (1993) Obesity and socioeconomic status—a complex relation. New Engl J Med 329:1036–1037
28. Rogers EM, Shoemaker EF (1971) Communication of innovation. Free Press, New York
29. Pietinen P, Nissinen A, Vartiainen E, Tuomilehto J, Uusitalo U, Ketola A, Moisio S, Puska P (1988) Dietary changes in the North Karelia Project (1972–1982). Prev Med 17:183–193

Discussion

Bangladeshi student: You indicate that smoking and body mass index are both rising in women at the same time that coronary death rates are declining. Can we conclude that if we can reduce cholesterol level we shouldn't worry at all about the other risk factors, including smoking?

J. Pekkanen: I would certainly not suggest anything like that. I agree with Dr. Beaglehole that we have to be cautious about interpreting these disease trends because their causal association with risk factors cannot be known. In Finland, blood pressure and cholesterol were so much stronger determinants of mortality in women, and the changes in them were so much larger than the changes in smoking, that those findings fit very well with the mortality trend in women.

J. Stamler: I would like to make a few comments about this fine series of papers and the very rich amount of data we have heard. My first is that the most difficult task we tackle in epidemiology is to relate trends of lifestyles and risk factors to trends on disease, mortality, and incidence. This is particularly true when we try to attribute percent changes in decline of the disease to x, y, or z factor. I usually refuse to try to do this and I share in the notes of caution expressed here. The coincidental findings are very encouraging, but we need to be cautious in their interpretation.

The second point is that it seems likely in my judgment that changes in nutrition are making a contribution to the decline in disease, independently of their impact on cholesterol and blood pressure, but we have so few data on cohorts to plug into the disease decline that we can't examine this. A similar situation exists in regard to alcohol consumption and physical activity, key aspects of lifestyle that are also related to trends, and we are also unable to plug these into trend analyses. This needs to be kept in mind.

Finally, when we look at these trends, we have to keep in mind that findings on adult cardiovascular disease risk factors and mortality can relate not only to patterns during adulthood but all the way back to fetal exposure and the first year of life. None of us has been able to plug any such variables into our adult analyses. The nearest we can come to such variables is the use of height as an index of early development. There may be something to the story that there is a conditioning of adult chronic disease, and cardiovascular disease risk, that begins as early as fetal life. This is interesting for science and public health and may be reflected in the differences found in social class trends. For all these reasons, we need to be cautious in relating adult trends in risk factors with trends in disease.

Part 4
Lessons from the Seven Countries Study

Will Measures to Prevent Coronary Heart Disease Protect Against Other Chronic Disorders?

Frederick H. Epstein

Summary. The possibility that coronary heart disease could be prevented was hardly considered until around 1950. The history of the developments which led to creating the scientific foundations for prevention, including the role played by the Seven Countries Study, is reviewed. There is now a need to move from cardiovascular disease prevention to the prevention of other major chronic disorders in order to reduce the total burden of chronic illness and mortality in individuals and the population at large. Evidence for links between cardiovascular and noncardiovascular diseases is summarized, suggesting that they share some common causes and may thus be amenable to the same preventive measures. These links include correlations between these groups of diseases within and between countries, similarities in the lifestyles predisposing to a number of chronic disorders, and demonstrations that the predictiveness of coronary disease risk-factors extends to other diseases. Furthermore, there is a correlation between the secular mortality trends for heart disease, cancer, stroke, and total mortality. The problems of devising all-encompassing chronic disease prevention strategies, as opposed to strategies directed to single diseases, are discussed. The Seven Countries Study, combining as it does the advantages of ecological comparisons and observations on cohorts, provides one model for new investigations into the potential of chronic disease prevention on a broad front.

Key words. Coronary heart disease—Chronic disease—Epidemiology—Prevention—Lifestyles—Mortality statistics—Risk factors—International comparisons

Introduction

The possibility of preventing a chronic disorder such as coronary heart disease has, it would seem, hardly been given a thought until around 1950. This seems strange, because the search for the causes of the underlying condition, atherosclerosis, dates back well into the last century, and the reason for

179

wanting to know the cause of a disease is surely the wish to treat and prevent it. One of the early visionaries was the great cardiologist Sir James Mackenzie, but the aim of the St. Andrews Study which he conceived in the early 1920s and could never complete was not so much the prevention as the early detection of coronary heart disease at a stage when its progression could be halted [1]. The history of coronary heart disease epidemiology as a deliberate and systematic science started in the late 1940s. The idea of prevention must have been in the mind of Ancel Keys, first and foremost, as well as the few other "founding fathers," but the first mention of the term *prevention* is in a publication of Keys in 1953 [2]. Even in the historic symposium on cardiovascular disease epidemiology at the Second World Congress of Cardiology a year later, organized by Keys and P.D. White, the word "prevention" was used only once and merely in passing by J.N. Morris [3]. In an important but hardly known paper by Keys, published in 1949, the emphasis was on long-term prediction, without mentioning prevention [4]. There was apparently a tacit assumption that it would be pointless to talk much about prevention before being firmly on the way toward the understanding of the disease and its precursors.

Some of this groundwork had been laid as early as 1956 at a symposium on the occasion of the annual meeting of the American Public Health Association, when serum cholesterol, blood pressure, and in part smoking were shown to be what were later to be called risk factors [5]. Around 1960, preventive trials started to be planned. A milestone along the way was Stamler's book, *Lectures on Preventive Cardiology*, published in 1967 [6]. One of the remarkable success stories of modern medicine has been unfolding so that, within the amazingly short span of 30 to 35 years, which is very short for a disease with such a long incubation period, coronary heart disease came to be by far the most powerfully predictable and potentially most preventable of all the chronic diseases. In addition, a model for the epidemiological study of other chronic disorders was created.

After this tour de force, it would not have been surprising if some degree of fatigue had set in. However, quite the contrary, the vitality of cardiovascular disease epidemiology is, if anything, still on the rise, as evidenced by the impressive program of the recent International Congress of Preventive Cardiology in Oslo (1993). There is no question that there is still much to be learned, while applying and putting into action the knowledge already in hand. There is a question, nevertheless, whether the spectacular vertical development toward greater heights of effective action and into greater depths of understanding needs to be paralleled by a horizontal expansion to other chronic disorders. Progress in medicine has been mostly in terms of categorical studies of separate diseases, as most of medical teaching addresses organ systems rather than whole human beings. Single diseases may have multiple causes and thus have a multifactorial etiology, like coronary heart disease. At the same time, single factors, such as smoking, may affect multiple organ systems and thus cause a variety of diseases. On the individual level, there may be, in addition, a general disease susceptibility so that illnesses cluster in the same people, explaining why there is a scale from people who always seem to be healthy to those who are always troubled by one or another disease. This translates, on the community level, to a relative minority of the population harboring a relative majority of the prevalent diseases for which we had some unpublished evidence in the Tecumseh Study of an entire community. While a general disease susceptibility of constitutional origin must be taken into account, the present focus is on causative factors with influences which transcend the borderlines between single diseases. The point of departure, therefore, is a lifestyle rather than a disease. Included are particularly dietary habits, smoking, physical activity, and psychosocial factors, all of which have, in all likelihood, simultaneous effects on multiple organs. Whatever the underlying reasons, these considerations open up the possibility that the measures which prevent coronary heart disease and related cardiovascular conditions could also protect health on a much broader front, not only prolonging life, but increasing the disability-free years with advancing age.

These considerations are not far removed from the Seven Countries Study and the long-term program of the Laboratory of Physiological Hygiene from which it originated. The ultimate concern is with health rather than disease, with physiology rather than pathology. The major interest, over the years, of the laboratory which Ancel Keys led to so much scientific distinction, happened to be the circulatory system, but the scope and outlook have always been larger, toward the "biology of man", part of the title of the important early paper quoted before [4]. Moreover, Keys' studies of mortality rates were never limited to coronary heart disease. The subtitle of the book on the Seven Countries Study is *A Multivariate Analysis of Death and Coronary Heart Disease* [7]. The book itself contains data on total deaths, coronary deaths, and noncoronary deaths, including deaths due to cancer, violence, accidents, and other causes. There are publications on an analysis of all deaths [8] and on the relations between diet and the all-cause death rate, including the important information on the correlations with monounsaturated fatty acids [9,10]. With regard to obesity, the relationship to longevity and total mortality was always included in the analyses [11]. It is clear that Keys' preoccupation was not only with the contribution of cardiac deaths to total deaths, but with noncardiac causes of death in their own right.

It may be asked why noncardiac diseases have been something of a stepchild in prospective studies of coronary heart disease. In part, there was probably some lack of interest. Another part was due to the problem of accurately diagnosing these other disorders. Last, but not least, the number of events was often insufficient for adequate statistical evaluation. The turning point came in 1981, at the time of the Workshop on Non-Cardiovascular Disease Mortality at the National Heart, Lung and Blood Institute in Bethesda [12], when the problem of the possible risk of low serum cholesterol on noncardiac diseases raised its head; it suddenly appeared that many prospective cardiovascular studies had valuable data on noncardiac mortality, as amply confirmed at a follow-up conference in 1990 [13]. A lot of regrettable damage was done to coronary heart disease prevention efforts by the concerns over the largely alleged risk of low serum cholesterol, but a secondary gain has been that much has been learned in the process about the relationships of coronary risk factors to noncardiovascular diseases. In addition, epidemiological interest in these interrelationships has been stimulated.

The Seven Countries Study is not only the first, but still the only cross-cultural epidemiological investigation which relates, by strictly comparable methods, both individual and population coronary heart disease risk to the mode of life and risk factors. It serves as a guide to extend this approach to other chronic diseases which, along with cardiac disorders, add up to the total burden of mortality and preceding morbidity. There is every reason to believe that the comparison of such relationships in populations with differing living conditions will provide insights, as in the Seven Countries Study, beyond those obtainable from single populations. These are perspectives for the future, building upon the evidence which is already available.

Interrelationships Between Chronic Diseases

There are several lines of evidence that cardiovascular and noncardiovascular disease mortality rates are correlated. The most impressive early data were published in the United States in 1959 [14], although the authors did not emphasize the finding. When cardiovascular and noncardiovascular death rates in the States of the Union are plotted against each other, a significant positive correlation is found. International comparisons show a lesser degree of association (unpublished observations), and in the Seven Countries Study there is no correlation between coronary deaths and deaths from other causes [7]. The difference of degree between within-country and between-country data requires explanation, but it stands to reason that the interrelationships among broad causes of death are more complex in cross-cultural settings. For more specific causes of death, such as ischemic heart disease and colorectal cancer, the correlation in 49 countries is as high as 0.74 [15]. It is most noteworthy that the secular decline of coronary heart disease mortality in the United States has attracted much more attention than the parallel finding of declines in mortality from each specific major cause of death except lung cancer and chronic lung disease [16].

It would be important to extend the mortality data to morbidity. In the Tecumseh Study, an early attempt was made to cross-relate the prevalence data for major chronic diseases [17]; the clustering of these diseases in individuals has already been mentioned. Clusters of illness and symptoms have been found in a community study in Israel [18].

Relationships of Coronary Heart Disease
Risk Factors to Other Diseases

Are coronary heart disease risk factors predictive for other diseases as well, which would again suggest that there is a sharing of common causes? Another early attempt in this direction was made in the Tecumseh Study [17]. A systematic study of this question was made for the first time some 10 years ago, using data from the Italian cohorts of the Seven Countries Study [19]. The most important finding was that the multiple logistic function, derived for coronary heart disease and including cholesterol, blood pressure, and smoking, was also predictive for other major causes of death and for total mortality. Recent unpublished data from the PROCAM Study in Germany likewise demonstrate that coronary heart disease and total mortality show a parallel increase in risk with rising multiple logistic function scores calculated for coronary disease (G. Assmann and H. Schulte, personal communication, 1993). A detailed analysis of the separate contributions to total mortality by the three risk factors indicates that blood pressure and smoking are uniformly predictive of all-cause mortality in six of the seven areas of the Seven Countries Study (the U.S. data were not available for this particular analysis) and in six large prospective studies in the United States; cholesterol, on the other hand, predicted total mortality in only two of the six American studies [20]. The data from the NRF Study in Rome further indicate that blood pressure and smoking are significantly predictive of coronary heart disease and cardiovascular and noncardiovascular disease, while the relationship with cholesterol is present for coronary and cardiovascular disease only [20]. It is to be expected that the relationship between cholesterol and noncardiovascular disease, as well as total mortality, is more complex than for blood pressure and smoking because it is influenced by confounding factors in the low cholesterol range [21]. All the above data refer to men only, since corresponding analyses have not been possible for women.

Summarizing the data on risk factors, blood pressure, and smoking are not only predictors of cardiovascular, but also other causes of mortality. The probability that cholesterol also contributes to noncardiovascular risk is by no means excluded, and would probably emerge if confounding factors at the lower end of the cholesterol distribution were taken into account. This interpretation is supported by the observation in the MRFIT Study that men with low cholesterol and blood pressure who do not smoke have less than half the total mortality of the whole cohort and a 30% lower cancer and 20% lower noncardiovascular, noncancer mortality, compared to the whole cohort [22]. Moreover, there are coronary risk factors other than cholesterol, blood pressure, and smoking, and the risk they carry may also extend to other diseases. Lastly, the analyses to date refer only to mortality, and the relationships to morbidity may conceivably be more pronounced.

Lifestyles and Chronic Diseases

If it could be shown that the lifestyles which predispose to cardiovascular diseases also add to the risk of other chronic disorders, it would constitute a direct demonstration that coronary heart disease prevention has beneficial consequences which are more far-reaching. A first suggestion in this direction came from the Alameda County Study in California. A "health practices index," which reflects seven daily habits along a scale from "healthy" to "unhealthy," correlated strongly not only with ischemic heart disease and other cardiovascular diseases, but with mortality from cancer and all other causes of death in both men and women. Grading the index into low, medium, and high, the relative mortality risk between low and high was of the order of threefold [23]. It is to be hoped that further evidence along these lines will come from the large community intervention projects now in progress. The demonstration of community effects for noncardiovascular diseases and total mortality takes a long time. In the North Karelia Project (P. Puska, unpublished data, 1993), it took 20 years until a definitive effect of intervention on cancer mortality could be shown. There are several reasons for these long periods of delay, one of them being that mortality from several causes is already declining in a number of countries so that intervention effects are more difficult to establish.

Further evidence that lifestyles affect several chronic diseases simultaneously comes from the Whitehall Study [24]. The civil servants in that study fall into four different social grades, total mortality being lowest in the highest grades. However, this social grade difference is present for each single cause of death, suggesting that the daily living habits within each grade have a large influence on health and disease over a broad range of illness. It is likely that access to medical care and its use are also related to the state of health in the different grades, but it is unlikely that the observed phenomenon is entirely or even largely due to better medical treatment for those in higher grades. On the other hand, it is likely that, among others, psychosocial factors are involved. There is much evidence that the work environment plays a role in coronary heart disease risk which may also extend to other conditions. For example, the strain caused by a job in which an employee is exposed to a high demand but has little power of decision may be deleterious. Job security may be protective. There are a good many theories, some well-supported, linking psychosocial factors to cardiovascular and probably to other diseases. The important point in the present context is that some of these factors are amenable to change.

The most pervasive and probably the most important lifestyle linking the risks of several chronic disorders is the habitual diet. In particular, dietary fat is related to atherosclerosis, some types of cancer, and diabetes. The evidence has been summarized in several recent publications [25–27]. As one example, the correlation between ischemic heart disease mortality and animal fat consumption for 33 countries is 0.55 for men and 0.24 for women (the gender difference may be related to differences in the secular trends between women and men); the corresponding correlations for cancer are 0.69 for men and 0.66

Table 1. Effects of lifestyles on chronic disease risk[a].

| | Atherosclerosis | | | |
	Heart disease	Stroke	Cancer	Diabetes
Diet[b]				
Body weight	3	3	3	3
Total fat	3	3	3	3
Fatty acid ratio	3	2	1	3
Fruits and vegetables	3	2	3	3
Complex carbohydrates	3	2	2	3
Antioxidants	2	1	1	2
Sodium (via blood pressure)	3	3	1	1
Calcium	1	1	1	1
Alcohol consumption	3	3	3	2
Smoking	3	3	3	3
Level of physical activity	3	1	2	3
Psychosocial factors	3	2	2	3

[a] Definite or probable, 3; likely, 2; possible, 1.
[b] Data from [25–27].

for women [28]. These are high correlations, particularly since no time lag has been taken into account.

The lifestyle factors which have been discussed can be summarized (Table 1). The strengths of the relationships with atherosclerotic diseases, cancer, and stroke have been arbitrarily graded on a scale from 1 to 3. The dietary components have been listed in detail, omitting selenium because it largely relates to the environment. Alcohol and physical activity [29] have been added. In general, the links provide hope that lifestyle changes toward the prevention of coronary heart disease would lead, in addition, to reducing the risk of other chronic disorders.

Secular Chronic Disease Mortality Trends

Against the background of the developments which have been described, it would be reasonable to expect that the secular trends in coronary heart disease mortality might be accompanied by corresponding trends in mortality from other major diseases. In contrast to the heart disease mortality trends, these other trends had received much less attention, and no attempt had been made to compare them with those from heart disease. A comprehensive analysis of the trends for total mortality and the main causes of death which contribute to it was carried out under the auspices of the National Heart, Lung and Blood Institute in Bethesda [30]. The monograph describes the trends for the separate causes of death and their interrelationships. Only the latter are under discussion in the present context and a summary of some of the findings will be

Table 2. Concordance of secular trends for mortality from coronary heart disease and cancer other than lung cancer for two age groups in 23 countries during two periods: 1950–1954 to 1965–1969 (I) and 1965–1969 to 1979–1983 (II).

	Number of concordant countries/ all countries	
	Age 45–64 years	Age 65–74 years
Men		
Contemporary analysis		
Period I	13/23	14/23
Period II	18/23	14/23
Time-lag analysis[a]	21/23 (91%)	19/23 (83%)
Women		
Contemporary analysis		
Period I	20/23	18/23
Period II	22/23	20/23
Time-lag analysis[a]	20/23 (87%)	20/23 (87%)

[a] Comparing CHD mortality during period I with mortality from cancer other than lung cancer during period II (15 years later).

shown. The methods used in the analysis and quantification of the trends are described in the monograph.

The most important comparison concerns the trends for heart disease and cancer. Since the trends for lung cancer have been upward in most countries until recently, cancer of the lung and other cancers have to be analyzed separately. When the secular trends for mortality from coronary heart disease and cancer other than lung cancer are tested for concordance in 23 countries between 1950 and 1983 in two time periods and two age groups in men, contemporary analysis indicates that there are more countries showing concordance than discordance, but the difference is not marked (Table 2). It is most likely, however, that heart disease mortality changes more rapidly in response to changes in the environment or lifestyles than cancer; the delayed response in cancer mortality has already been pointed out in connection with the North Karelia Study. If a time lag of 15 years is assumed (Table 2), a striking degree of concordance emerges in the case of both younger and older men. For women, the trends are mostly concordant even on contemporary analysis, reflecting the universal tendency toward a secular decline of mortality in women.

For heart disease versus lung cancer trends (Table 3) in 27 countries, there is a surprising degree of concordance in men during the two time periods, with a tendency to increase on time-lag analysis. This degree of concordance would not have been expected, because the secular trends for the two diseases are opposite in many countries, but it makes sense in view of the common link with

Table 3. Concordance of secular trends for mortality from coronary heart disease and lung cancer for two age groups during two periods: 1950–1954 to 1965–1969 (I) and 1965–1969 to 1979–1983 (II).

	Number of concordant countries/ all countries	
	Ages 45–64 years	Ages 65–74 years
Men		
Contemporary analysis		
Period I	17/27	17/27
Period II	13/27	10/27
Time-lag analysis[a]	18/26 (69%)	20/26 (77%)
Women		
Contemporary analysis		
Period I	2/27	4/27
Period II	4/27	5/27
Time-lag analysis[a]	3/26 (11.5%)	3/26 (11.5%)

[a] Comparing CHD mortality during period I with mortality from cancer during period II (15 years later).

Table 4. Concordance of secular trends for mortality from coronary heart disease and cerebrovascular disease for two age groups during two periods: 1950–1954 to 1965–1969 (I) and 1965–1969 to 1979–1983 (II).

	Number of concordant countries/ all countries	
	Ages 45–64 years	Ages 65–74 years
Men		
Contemporary analysis		
Period I	7/27	12/27
Period II	23/27 (85%)	20/27 (74%)
Women		
Contemporary analysis		
Period I	19/27	18/27
Period II	21/27 (78%)	24/27 (89%)

smoking. The total lack of concordance in women (Table 3) is anticipated on account of the almost universal decline of heart disease trends, in contrast to lung cancer trends. Coronary heart disease and cerebrovascular disease mortality trends show much concordance in men during the second time period and in women, even on contemporary analysis; there is no reason for assuming a time lag in this instance (Table 4). The results of these analyses are encouraging in lending support to the hypothesis which has been proposed.

There is no claim that these secular trend analyses are, at this stage, persuasive in themselves. They are merely, so far, tending to be in line with other evidence, also still no more than strongly suggestive, that coronary heart disease prevention holds a major key toward the prevention of other chronic disorders as well. The evidence needs strengthening on all the levels which have been discussed, seeking, in addition, other approaches. As far as secular trend analyses are concerned, the data presented need extension to longer time periods and, especially, to an analysis in terms of specific types of cancer.

Future Strategies

There is always a question when scientific evidence is strong enough to act upon it at the public health and individual level. Action to prevent coronary heart disease will move forward, despite the obstacles still being put in the way. If the hypothesis proposed is correct, the strategies to prevent coronary disease would, without any additional effort, have the prevention of other disorders, so to speak, as a by-product. It should be asked, however, whether health promotion campaigns geared toward the preservation of health in broad terms rather than toward the prevention of any specific disease might be more effective. This cannot by any means be taken for granted and depends, apart from presumably other considerations, on whether health messages referring directly to heart disease, or for that matter to cancer, are more readily intelligible and acceptable than what might seem vague appeals to preserve general health. Even in the best cardiovascular community education projects, the effect on risk factors, especially in the case of serum cholesterol, falls short of the desirable target levels [31]. There is apparently still room for improving the currently used methods of motivation in heart disease prevention programs. More broadly conceived chronic disease prevention programs, with the emphasis on the preservation of health in general, would clearly require new orientations with regard to encouraging motivation for a change toward more healthy lifestyles. The question is raised for consideration, without proposing answers.

There is another aspect to noncategorical disease prevention programs. At the present time, there are no cancer or diabetes prevention and control programs which can compare with the intense efforts of national and community levels in the area of cardiovascular disease prevention. There is a need, however, to step up prevention programs for all chronic diseases with a potential for prevention. It would clearly be wasteful and inefficient to launch campaigns for each of these disorders separately, and people in the population would resent being exposed to parallel and uncoordinated demands on their attention [32]. Coordinated, comprehensive programs constitute the only realistic approach. In this connection, the important and essential role of practicing physicians to participate in preventive efforts must be recalled.

The World Health Organization has recognized the need for integrated prevention and control of noncommunicable diseases [33]. After several exploratory meetings, a formal WHO conference took place in Kaunas in 1981 [34]. Since that time, the Interhealth Programme [33] has come into being, aiming to carry out demonstration projects in several developing and developed countries. These international activities are essential and encouraging, but there is also a need for individual countries to further these trends on their own initiative.

Epilogue

This symposium is concerned with the lessons for science from the Seven Countries Study. Preventive cardiology would not have developed into one of the remarkable success stories in modern medicine, as stated in the beginning, if there had not been a tremendous and dedicated effort on the part of many investigators and organizations all over the world. The entire body of knowledge and action adds up to much more than the sum of the individual contributions. For this and other reasons, it would be idle to partition the contributions in order of their importance. There is no doubt, however, that some links in the chain of evidence are much stronger than others, and there are few, if any, single links as strong as the Seven Countries Study. Without it, the evidence that cross-cultural differences in coronary heart disease risk are closely tied to the major risk factors would be almost entirely based on ecological comparisons. It is true that there are a good many studies in several countries which have related risk factors to risk, but they cannot be compared with any degree of reliability because of differences in methodology. This is not to belittle the importance of ecological comparisons. Quite the contrary, they are of the greatest value as long as their limitations are recognized, including the fact that they do not always provide the same information as observations on cohorts [35]. The Seven Countries Study has all the advantages of ecological comparisons without their disadvantages because the simultaneous availability of cohort data permits mutual verification.

Whenever there has been much achievement, the journey should not stop but continue. The Seven Countries Study has not only yielded scientific data, but it has created an epidemiological model for field studies which might be used for approaching other problems. Certainly, the model should serve for further intensive investigations of cardiovascular diseases. The implication of all that has been said so far in this presentation is to propose to use this model, in addition, for the study of interrelationships between chronic diseases, with the aim toward their prevention as a whole. An attempt was made to review the admittedly preliminary evidence to date that the cardiovascular diseases share with other major chronic disorders a number of common causes so that the preventive potential of lifestyle changes thought to relate primarily to coronary heart disease would be greatly enhanced. It is reasonable to think that studies patterned after the model of the Seven Countries Study, looking at risk and risk-factor constellations cross-culturally, will yield new clues on the determinants of chronic disease frequency and life expectation. In connection with this search, it must be remembered how fortunate it was, in the case of coronary heart disease, that the hypotheses as regards predisposing factors which existed in the late 1940s could be confirmed; the present situation with regard to factors predisposing to cancer would seem to be less clearly defined and this applies as well to some of the other noncardiovascular chronic disorders. Clues on causes do not come, of course, from epidemiological observations alone, but the chances are that international comparisons between countries with higher and lower disease frequencies will provide new insights.

The concept of international comparisons as part of epidemiological research is not new but goes back, under the name of "geographical pathology," well into the last century. However, essentially all of these studies used already existing data, particularly mortality statistics. The idea of carrying out collaborative and coordinated field studies in different countries, deliberately designed to answer specific questions, was entirely novel and, in fact, like so many of Ancel Keys' ideas, revolutionary. This approach ought to serve well to address some of the questions which have been asked in this chapter. It should lead to achieving not only the prevention of clinical disease and premature death, but the preservation of disability-free years with advancing age. This would be progress from geographical pathology to geographical hygiene, in the sense of the term "physiological hygiene" which has guided Ancel Keys' life work.

References

1. MacKenzie J (1926) The basis of vital activity: being a review of five years' work at the St. Andrews Institute for Clinical Research. Faber and Gwyer, London
2. Keys A (1953) Prediction and possible prevention of coronary disease. Am J Publ Health 43:1399–1407
3. Keys A, White PD (eds) (1956) Cardiovascular epidemiology. Paul B Hoeber, New York
4. Keys A (1949) The physiology of the individual as an approach to a more quantitative biology of man. Fed Proc 8:523–529
5. Measuring the risk of coronary heart disease in adult populations—a symposium. Am J Publ Health 47[Suppl I]:1–63
6. Stamler J (1967) Lectures on preventive cardiology. Grune and Stratton, New York
7. Keys A, Aravanis C, Blackburn, H, Buzina R, Djordjevic B, Dontas A, Fidanza F, Karvonen M, Kimura N, Menotti A, Mohacek I, Nedeljkovic S, Puddu V, Punsar S, Taylor H, van Buchem FSP (1980) Seven Countries Study: a multivariate analysis of death and coronary heart disease. Harvard University Press, Cambridge, Mass.
8. Keys A, Menotti A, Aravanis C, Blackburn H, Djordjevic BS, Buzina R, Dontas AS, Fidanza F, Karvonen MJ, Kimura N, Mohacek I, Nedeljkovic S, Puddu V, Punsar S, Taylor HL, Conti S, Kromhout D, Toshima H (1984) The seven countries study: 2289 deaths in 15 years. Prev Med 13:2141–154

9. Keys A, Aravanis C, van Buchem FSP, Blackburn H, Buzina R, Djordjevic BS, Dontas AS, Fidanza F, Karvonen MJ, Kimura N, Menotti A, Nedeljkovic S, Puddu V, Punsar S, Taylor HL (1981) The diet and all-cause death rate in the Seven Countries Study. Lancet 2:58–61

10. Keys A, Menotti A, Karvonen MJ, Aravanis C, Blackburn H, Buzina R, Djordjevic BS, Dontas AS, Fidanza F, Keys MH, Kromhout D, Nedeljkovic S, Punsar S, Seccareccia F, Toshima H (1986) The diet and 15-year death rate in the Seven Countries study. Am J Epidemiol 124:903–915

11. Keys A (1992) Longevity and body fatness in middle age. Nutr Metab Cardiovasc Dis 2:11–18

12. Feinleib M (1982) Summary of a workshop on cholesterol and non-cardiovascular disease mortality. Prev Med 11:360–367

13. Jacobs D, Blackburn H, Higgins M, Reed D, Iso H, McMillan GC, Neaton J, Nelson J, Potter J, Rifkind B, Rossouw J, Shekelle R, Yusuf S (1992) Report of a conference on low blood cholesterol: mortality associations. Circulation 86: 1046–1060

14. Sauer HI, Enterline PE (1959) Are geographic variations in death rates from cardiovascular disease real? J Chronic Dis 10:513–524

15. Sidney S, Farquhar JW (1983) Cholesterol, cancer and public health policy. Am J Med 75:494–508

16. Thom TJ, Kannel WB, Feinleib M (1958) Factors in the decline of coronary heart disease mortality. In: Connor WE, Bristow JD (eds) Coronary heart disease—prevention, complications, treatment. Lippincott, Philadelphia, pp 5–20

17. Epstein FH, Francis T Jr, Hayner NS, Johnson BC, Kjelsberg MO, Napier JA, Ostrander LD Jr, Payne MW, Dodg HJ (1965) Prevalence of chronic diseases and distribution of selected physiologic variables in a total community, Tecumseh, Michigan. Am J Epidemiol 81:307–322

18. Abramson JH, Gofin J, Peritz E, Hopp C, Epstein LM (1981) Clustering of chronic disorders—a community study of coprevalence in Jerusalem. J Chronic Dis 35: 221–230

19. Menotti A, Conti S, Dima F, Giampaoli S, Giuli B, Rumi A, Seccareccia F, Signoretti P (1983) Prediction of all causes of death as a function of some factors commonly measured in cardiovascular disease surveys. Prev Med 12:318–325

20. Menotti A (1992) Coronary risk factors and non-cardiovascular disease. In: Marmot M, Elliott P (eds) Coronary heart disease epidemiology. From aetiology to public health. Oxford University Press, Oxford, pp 298–310

21. Epstein FH (1992) Low cholesterol cancer and other non-cardiovascular disorders. Atherosclerosis 94:1–12

22. Stamler J, Dyer AR, Shekelle RB, Neaton J, Stamler R (1993) Relationship of baseline major risk factors to coronary and all-cause mortality, and to longevity: findings from long-term follow-up of Chicago cohorts. Cardiology 82:191–222

23. Wingard DL, Berkman LF, Brand RJ (1982) A multivariate analysis of health-related practices: a nine year mortality follow-up of the Alameda County Study. Am J Epidemiol 116:765–775

24. Marmot MG, Shipley MJ, Rose G (1984) Inequalities in death-specific explanations of a general pattern. Lancet 1:1003–1006

25. Committee on Diet and Health, Food and Nutrition Board, Commission on Life Sciences, National Research Council (1989) Diet and health—implications for reducing chronic disease risk. National Academy Press, Washington, D.C.

26. Report of a WHO Study Group (1990) Diet, nutrition, and the prevention of chronic diseases. World Health Organization Technical Report Series 797, World Health Organization, Geneva
27. Waldron KW, Johnson IT, Fenwick GR (eds) (1993) Food and cancer prevention: chemical and biological aspects. Royal Society of Chemistry, Cambridge
28. Kesteloot H (1992) Nutrition and health. Eur Heart J 13:120–128
29. Paffenbarger RS, Hyde RT, Wing AL, Lee I-M, Jung DL, Kampert JB (1993) The association of changes in physical activity level and other lifestyle characteristics with mortality among men. N Engl J Med 328:538–545
30. Thom TJ, Epstein FH, Feldman JJ, Leaverton PE, Wolz M (1992) Total mortality and mortality from heart disease, cancer and stroke from 1950 to 1987 in 27 countries—highlights of trends and their interrelationships among causes of death. National Institutes of Health, National Heart, Lung and Blood Institute, NIH publication no 92-3088, Bethesda, Md.
31. Fortmann SP, Taylor CB, Flora JA, Winkleby MA (1993) Effect of community health education on plasma cholesterol levels and diet: the Stanford Five-City Project. Am J Epidemiol 137:1039–1055
32. Epstein FH, Holland WW (1983) Prevention of chronic diseases in the community— one disease versus multiple disease strategies. Int J Epidemiol 12:135–137
33. Interhealth Steering Committee (1991) Demonstration projects for the integrated prevention and control of non-communicable diseases (Interhealth Programme): epidemiological background and rationale. World Health Statist Q 44:48–54
34. Glasunov IS, Grabauskas V, Holland WW, Epstein FH (1983) An integrated programme for the prevention and control of non-communicable diseases. J Chronic Dis 36:419–426
35. Blackburn H, Jacobs D (1984) Sources of the diet—heart controversy: confusion over population versus individual correlations. Circulation 70:775–780

Discussion

A. Keys: I should like to point out that what we have heard from Fred Epstein goes back a long time. While I was on sabbatical at Oxford a very long time ago (1950–51), I attended a nutrition conference in Rome where I wanted to talk about coronary heart disease while the delegates assembled wanted to talk about dietary deficiencies. Professor Bergami of Naples explained that "we have no coronary problem in Italy."

So, I proceeded to find out whether this was true or not. We found, indeed, that there was a reason for Bergami's remarks. There was almost no coronary disease in the general population, but cases were seen among the wealthier classes, along with an enormous difference in lifestyle. We made the same kind of study several months later in Madrid with the same answers about social class differences.

Shortly afterward, I was invited to lecture in Amsterdam at a joint meeting on diabetes and nutrition attended by more than 1000 investigators. I don't believe that 10 of them believed there was anything in what I was saying! In contrast, some months later I gave the same lecture to a very small audience in

New York and one person in that small audience *was* interested! He became a "disciple" to the idea and spread the word far better than I could, influencing the opinions of people all over the world. That person was Fred Epstein.

F. Epstein: Thank you very much, Ancel. And look at me now!

R. Beaglehole: Thank you, Professor Epstein, for your stimulating address. I wonder if you would comment on the likelihood of success on the point with which you ended, in regard to avoidable ill health and disability. Are we doing well in terms of longevity and quality of life?

F. Epstein: I have been talking about disability for years. One wonders whether preventing these chronic diseases will necessarily lead not only to longer life, but to a better and healthier life. There is now an international coordinated study going on trying to relate longevity in different countries to survey findings on morbidity, which I find an exciting and important idea. I think it is quite feasible in different countries with different degrees of longevity, to see whether in countries where people live longer, they have in effect less disability. This seems to be the case with preliminary data I have seen, and this makes an awful lot of sense. If healthier lifestyles prevent many diseases, they would also contribute to preserving health as well. It is one of the foremost tasks of our time, in an aging population, to provide evidence that this is, in fact, so.

R. Buzina: Dr. Epstein, your views have already taken form in WHO and FAO programs for health promotion. We are talking now not separately of cardiovascular disease or cancer, but about diet-related, noncommunicable diseases including cancer, cardiovascular diseases, gallstones, arthritis, and so on. On the other hand, for intervention methods we are combining the programs on lifestyle components, which automatically include all the risk factors and behaviors that influence them.

At the international nutrition conference in Rome last December, organized by WHO-FAO for policy makers and ministers of health and agriculture, these programs were accepted. We hope that this will be a useful strategy for the most important issues in developing countries now, that is, diet-related, chronic diseases. We hope that these components will become more and more integrated along the lines that you have suggested here.

The Potential for Prevention of the Major Adult Cardiovascular Diseases

JEREMIAH STAMLER

The Potential for Prevention: Scientific Foundation and Public Policy

This chapter deals with two aspects of the potential for prevention of cardiovascular disease: first, scientific data documenting this potential, emphasizing not high risk, but *low risk*; and second, public policy issues that relate to achievement of the potential for prevention. There are two aspects to the potential for prevention: one, the scientific foundation, the other, the comprehension of this by political leaders, the public, and the health professions, resulting in the translation of that potential into public policy and finally the implementation of that public policy [1].

The Scientific Foundation

National Trends in Diet and Coronary Heart Disease Mortality

Figure 1 shows results of recent 26-country ecologic analyses of Food and Agriculture Organization–World Health Organization (FAO–WHO) data. The FAO food balance sheets from 1961 to 1981 were converted to per capita mean nutrient intake by Dr. Marilyn Buzzard and her colleagues at the Nutrition Coordinating Center, University of Minnesota. Figure 1 shows the relationship between the 1961–1981 slope of dietary cholesterol and the 1972–1982 slope of age-standardized CHD mortality for men aged 40–69 years [2]. Similar data are available for the slope of percent calories from dietary saturated fatty acids (S) and for the slope of Keys score. These data deal with the relationship between *change* in the nutritional variable and *change* in coronary mortality, in which the correlation coefficient for the relationship of these two slopes is 0.83 for dietary cholesterol and CHD, 0.76 for saturates and CHD, 0.85 for Keys score and CHD, and no relationship for polyunsaturates and CHD ($r = -0.001$). The decline from 1961 to 1981 in national per capita

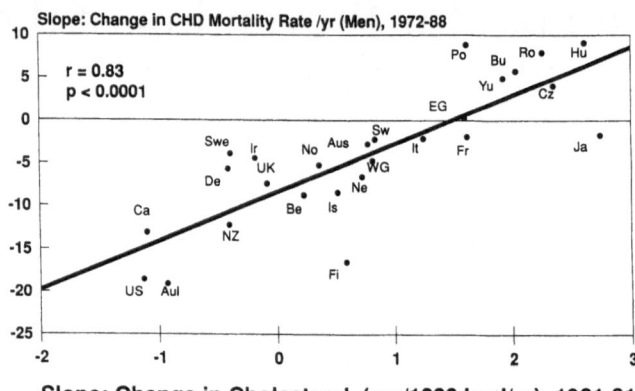

Fig. 1. Cross-population (ecologic) analysis of relationship between linear slope of national per capita dietary cholesterol (mg/1000 kcal per year), 1961–1981, and linear slope of age-standardized national coronary heart disease (CHD) mortality rate, 1972–1988, men ages 40–69 years, 26 countries. Dietary cholesterol data were derived from national food balance sheets from the Food and Agriculture Organization, Rome, Italy; age-sex-cause-specific mortality data, from the World Health Organization, Geneva, Switzerland. *US*, United States; *Ca*, Canada; *Aul*, Australia; *De*, Denmark; *NZ*, New Zealand; *Swe*, Sweden; *Ir*, Ireland; *UK*, United Kingdom; *Be*, Belgium; *No*, Norway; *Is*, Israel; *Fi*, Finland; *Aus*, Austria; *Ne*, the Netherlands; *WG*, West Germany; *Sw*, Switzerland; *It*, Italy; *EG*, East Germany; *Fr*, France; *Po*, Poland; *Yu*, Yugoslavia; *Bu*, Bulgaria; *Ro*, Romania; *Cz*, Czechoslovakia; *Hu*, Hungary; *Ja*, Japan. (Data from [2])

dietary cholesterol was associated with a decline in CHD mortality rate in many countries; for six eastern European countries, rise in dietary cholesterol was associated with increase in mortality from CHD.

Within-population Prospective Data on Major Risk Factors and Long-term Mortality Risks

Data within populations show the force of the relationship of serum cholesterol and other major risk factors to disease risk not only for middle-aged men, but also for older and younger persons.

Studies of Young Adult Men. Table 1 shows the relationship of baseline serum total cholesterol (TC) (one value per man) to age-standardized 19-year mortality from coronary heart disease (CHD), all cardiovascular diseases (CVD), all non-CVD causes, cancers, violence, other causes, and all causes for 11 139 men aged 18–39 years at baseline in the Chicago Heart Association Detection Project in Industry (CHA) Study [3]. Note the strength of the TC–CHD and TC–CVD relationships—a much steeper slope than that re-

Table 1. Baseline serum cholesterol and 19-year age-adjusted mortality by cause in 11 139 men ages 18–39 years at baseline, Chicago Heart Association Study. (a) deaths, (b) age-adjusted rate per 10 000 person-years.

Serum cholesterol level (mg/dl)	Number	Person-years	Mortality												
			CHD		CVD		Non-CVD		Cancer		Violent		Other		All	
			(a)	(b)	(a)	(b)	(a)	(b)	(a)	(b)	(a)	(b)	(a)	(b)	(a)	(b)
<160	2140	39 723	2	0.9	5	2.1	33	10.2	10	3.8	15	3.7	8	2.6	38	12.3
160–199	4826	89 207	19	2.2	32	3.7	116	13.4	39	4.6	48	5.4	29	3.3	148	17.1
200–239	3183	58 728	47	7.2	56	8.5	74	11.6	30	4.3	26	4.5	18	2.9	130	20.1
≥240	990	18 292	25	12.2	31	16.2	36	22.2	23	10.8	6	5.5	7	5.9	67	38.4

CHD, coronary heart disease; CVD, cardiovascular diseases.

Table 2. Proportional hazards regression coefficients for the relationship of multiple variables measured at baseline to 19-year risk of coronary, cardiovascular, and all–causes mortality, 11 139 men ages 18–39 years at baseline, Chicago Heart Association Study.

Variable[a]	Multivariate Cox regression coefficient		
	CHD death	CVD death	All-causes death
Serum cholesterol (mg/dl)	0.015546***	0.012745***	0.006583***
Systolic blood pressure (mmHg)	0.017732**	0.022932***	0.011644***
Cigarettes/day	0.029174***	0.027183***	0.025316***
Diabetes (yes, no)	1.580304***	1.300118***	0.900603**
Body mass index (kg/m^2)	−0.020007	−0.023384	−0.028725***
BMI^2	0.000036	0.000037	0.000049***
Education (years)	−0.092412*	−0.090546*	−0.122132***
Black (yes, no)	−0.688119	−0.450931	0.530685***
Other ethnicity (yes, no)	0.241385	−0.066093	−0.162646
Age (years)	0.085406***	0.083024***	0.061599***
Number of deaths	93	124	383

* $P < 0.05$; ** $P < 0.01$; *** $P < 0.001$.
[a] Other variables in analyses: former smoker, major ECG abnormalities, minor ECG abnormalities.

corded for middle-aged or older men. Note that the relative risk of CHD death for men with entry TC < 200 mg/dl is only one-eighth that of men with TC 200–239 mg/dl and only 7% that of men with TC ≥ 240 mg/dl. The multivariate Cox regression coefficient for TC–CHD was 0.0155 (Table 2), more than double the size of the coefficient for middle-aged men for this cohort and for several other cohorts, including those for Seven Countries Study men (0.0068 for U.S. railroad men, 0.0062 for northern European men, 0.0069 for southern European men, with 15-year follow-up) [4]. Based on the multivariate Cox coefficient, a TC lower by 40 mg/dl led to a relative risk of 0.538 (i.e., a risk lower by 46%) in the CHA Study. Similar findings were recorded with 25-year follow-up of the cohort of young adult men ages 25–39 years at baseline from the Chicago Peoples Gas (PG) Study [5].

Since all these estimates are based on a single determination of TC for each man, they are underestimates due to regression-dilution bias. Thus, for the cohort of Johns Hopkins medical students with multiple determinations of TC while they were at school, across quartiles of serum cholesterol (mean TC values 158, 181, 197, and 231 mg/dl), with up to 40 years of follow-up, rates of first major coronary events were 6.9, 11.5, 17.5, and 35.2 per 100 [6]. These data, free of the problem of regression-dilution bias, indicate that on average, for each 1% higher serum TC level there was a more than 5% higher long-term individual risk of a first major coronary event. This is a much greater increment in risk with higher TC than that often cited for middle-aged men, for example, 1% to 2%, based on prospective findings from the Framingham Study [7]; from the cohort of about 350 000 U.S. middle-aged men screened for the Multiple

Risk Factor Intervention Trial (MRFIT) [8]; and from results of the Lipid Research Clinics Coronary Primary Prevention Trial (LRC–CPPT) [9,10]. These data on young adult men demonstrate the great potential for CVD prevention with low serum TC in youth and young adulthood, and underscore the value of dietary patterns that preserve such levels into middle and older age.

Note, too, in Table 1 that for the young adult CHA cohort, entry serum TC level was directly related to risk of death from non-CVD causes, cancers, and other medical causes. There was no evidence among the large subset with low TC (< 160 mg/dl) of any adverse consequences. Further, TC did not relate significantly to risk of death from violent causes. Again, similar results were recorded for the cohort of Johns Hopkins medical students. These data on generally healthy young adults, in the labor force or attending medical school, along with similar findings for cohorts of generally healthy middle-aged persons, lend substantial support to the inference that for cohorts showing low TC to be associated with certain specific higher risks (e.g., for lung cancer and chronic obstructive pulmonary disease (COPD) in smokers, liver cirrhosis and liver cancer, hemorrhagic stroke), low TC is a marker for other problems and not in itself a cause of excess mortality risk [11,12]. Thus, low TC in youth and young adulthood, especially when maintained by favorable lifestyles over ensuing decades, not only predicts high potential for CHD and CVD prevention, but also for greater longevity with health. These findings are in accord with both the cross-population and within-population results of the Seven Countries Study on the critical role of serum cholesterol in CHD risk for populations and for individuals.

As was the case for three Seven Countries Study cohorts, for the CHA young adult men, cigarette use and blood pressure also were related to 19-year risk of CHD, CVD, and all-causes death [3]. The Cox coefficient for the relationship of cigarettes per day to CHD was 0.0292, so that the relative risk for nonsmokers compared to half-pack a day smokers was 0.747, that is, risk was 25% lower. The coefficient for the systolic blood pressure (SBP)–CHD relationship was 0.0177, so that the relative risk for a cohort with a mean SBP of 115 mmHg was 0.702 (30% lower) compared to a cohort with a mean SBP of 135 mmHg. These relative risks are multiplicative, so that for a cohort of men ages 18–39 with a mean TC of 160 mg/dl and a mean SBP of 115 mmHg, nonsmoking, compared to a cohort with the actual mean levels recorded for the CHA men ages 18–39 at entry (TC 190 mg/dl, SBP 135 mmHg, 10 cigarettes/day), the estimated relative risk was $0.627 \times 0.702 \times 0.747 = 0.329$, that is, a relative risk of CHD death during 19 years—from mean age 30 to mean age 49—lower by 67%.

Based on the coefficients for the relationship of the above three major risk factors to all-causes mortality, and for age and this end point, an estimate can be made of the impact of more favorable TC, SBP, and smoking status on longevity, again cohort mean TC of 160 mg/dl (instead of 190), SBP of 115 mmHg (instead of 135), and no cigarette use (instead of 10/day). Relative risks for all-causes death are 0.821 with 30 mg/dl lower TC; 0.792 with 20 mmHg lower SBP; 0.776 with no cigarette use (vs 10/day): 0.821 × 0.792 × 0.776 = 0.504 together, a 50% lower risk of death over the 19-year age span from mean age 30 to mean age 49 years. As to life expectancy, this translates into 2.9 additional years attributable to lower TC, 3.4 additional years due to lower SBP, and 3.8 additional years due to nonsmoking (vs 10/day)—altogether 10.1 years. (For the statistical procedure for use of Cox coefficients to estimate effects on longevity, see [5], pp 194 and 209–210.) Thus, instead of an expectation of 42.8 additional years, to age 72.8, for an average U.S. male aged 30 years [13], 42.8 + 10.1 = 52.9 additional years are estimated, to age 82.9 years. These are impressive potentials, not only for CHD–CVD prevention, but also for longer life with health. These data underscore the importance of primary prevention of the major risk factors themselves, through improved lifestyles, as the key to ending the CHD–CVD epidemic. This point is further supported by autopsy studies, including those in young adulthood, showing that atherogenesis begins in childhood and youth and also at that stage is related to risk factors, as shown, for example, by the PDAY study [14].

Dietary Variables and the Problem of Regression-dilution Bias. In regard to the major risk factors shown in Table 2 (serum TC, SBP, cigarettes per day, diabetes), cardiovascular epidemiology was "lucky"—ratios of intra- to interindividual variances were low, well under 1.0, so that it was possible to classify individuals within a population with adequate precision, albeit with some misclassification, so that the true association with CHD–CVD was always underestimated based on only one measurement (regression-dilution bias [15]). The situation is very different in regard to dietary variables, as Ancel Keys pointed out years ago [16]. For these, the ratio of intra- to interindividual variances is greater than 1.00. Hence with data from one 24-h dietary recall, considerable misclassification of individuals occurs. Regression coefficients of CHD on dietary cholesterol, S, and Keys score or of BP on dietary Na, K, protein, and lipids are driven toward zero [17]. Observed coefficients are routinely much below 50% of true coefficients [18,19]. False-negative findings are often the consequence, even with a carefully collected 24-h recall on each person. For years, failure to realize this problem—recently termed "regression-dilution bias" [15]—created confusion in CVD epidemiology, leading to the erroneous assertion that for individuals within populations, dietary lipid did not relate to either serum TC or CHD risk, despite unequivocal evidence from metabolic ward, cross-population, human intervention, and animal experimental studies that this was not correct.

Dietary Cholesterol-lipid and Mortality Risks of Middle-aged Men. This issue was set straight in the 1980s, particularly with publication of 19-year follow-up data from the Chicago Western Electric (WE) Study [20]. In that study, led by Oglesby Paul, an in-depth interview of every man was done at baseline and again 1 year later by a skilled nutritionist taking more than an hour per man to assess usual eating pattern in the previous 28 days (the Burke method) [21].

With this method, dietary lipid intake (Keys score) and particularly dietary cholesterol intake related to risks of death from CHD, CVD, and all causes significantly and independently of the other major risk factors. Data with 24-year follow-up are available (Table 3) [5,22]. Note that these are multivariate (Cox) analyses; all these factors are in the analyses together. The question being asked is *not* do dietary lipids influence serum lipids; that question was really answered years ago, as further validated in the WE baseline data. The question being asked here is, do dietary lipids relate to long-term mortality, *in addition to any effects they may have on serum cholesterol* and possibly also on systolic blood pressure (see below). The answer for dietary cholesterol is yes. Further analyses showed that dietary cholesterol related significantly to long-term mortality risk for subgroups of the WE men stratified into tertiles of entry serum TC. Daan Kromhout subsequently published similar data from Zutphen, The Netherlands, as have our colleagues in the Boston–Ireland Study and the Honolulu Heart Study, and there are also concordant data from food frequency studies of civil servants in The Netherlands and of Seventh Day Adventists in California [23]. Thus, this relationship can be regarded as well-established even though the mechanism is unclear—possible effects on lipoprotein fractions over and above effects on total serum cholesterol, possible effects on thrombogenic factors, etc. Whatever the mechanisms, the data show an independent effect of nutrition, particularly dietary cholesterol, on mortality risks.

As shown by estimates of relative risk and impact on longevity, this relationship is quantitatively important in regard to the potential for prevention (Table 3). Thus, a daily dietary cholesterol intake of 100 mg/1000 Kcal instead of 237 mg/1000 Kcal (as observed for the WE men) yields an estimate of 24-year CHD mortality relative risk of 0.681 (32% lower), and all-causes mortality risk of 0.822 (18% lower), translating into an estimated 2.0 years of greater life expectancy. Note also the favorable independent effects of a lower serum TC and SBP, and of nonsmoking, and the estimated combined multiplicative effects on relative risk and additive effects on longevity of favorable status for all four of these major risk factors: relative risk of 24-year CHD death 0.311 (69% lower) and all-causes death 0.434 (57% lower), and an estimated 8.6 years added to life expectancy (3.3 of these years from lower dietary cholesterol intake plus lower serum TC). Thus, for a 49-year old man (mean age of the WE cohort at baseline), instead of an expected 26.1 years of additional life on average to age 75.1 years, there is an expectation of 34.7 years, to age 83.7.

A similar comparison, of a cohort with all four lifestyle and lifestyle-related risk factors favorable (Table 3), compared to a higher-risk subcohort of WE men (diet cholesterol 400 mg/1000 Kcal, serum cholesterol 280 mg/dl, SBP 162 mmHg, cigarettes/day 20) yields these further estimates [5]: relative risk of 24-year CHD death 0.072 (93% lower) and all-causes death 0.145 (85% lower), and longevity greater by 20.5 years. Of those estimated 20.5 years, 4.5 are attributable to habitual lower intake of dietary cholesterol; 2.3 to lower serum

Table 3. Proportional hazards regression coefficients[a] for coronary heart disease and all-causes mortality, and estimated relative risks and longer years of life expectancy with favorable levels compared with baseline observed levels of four major risk factors, 24-year follow-up, 1882 white men ages 41–57 years at baseline in 1959, Western Electric Study.

Baseline variable	Coefficient		Favorable level	Observed level[b]	Relative risk[c]		Estimated years of greater life expectancy[d]
	CHD death	All death			CHD death	All death	
Dietary cholesterol (mg/1000 Kcal)	0.0028***	0.0014*	100	237	0.681	0.822	2.0
Serum cholesterol (mg/dl)	0.0055***	0.0024**	190	242	0.751	0.882	1.3
Systolic BP (mmHg)	0.0191***	0.0160***	118	132	0.766	0.799	2.3
Cigarettes/day	0.0230***	0.0289***	0	10	0.794	0.749	3.0
Age (years)	0.0519***	0.0823	44	49	0.771	0.663	4.3e
Deaths (n)	308	682					

* $P < 0.05$; ** $P < 0.01$; *** $P < 0.001$.

[a] Also in multivariate analyses: past smoker (no, yes), alcohol intake (ml/day), past drinker (no, yes), body mass index (kg/m^2), heart rate (beats/min), major ECG abnormality (no, yes), minor ECG abnormality (no, yes), diet saturated fat (% Kcal), diet polyunsaturated fat (% Kcal).

[b] Baseline mean value for whole cohort of 1882 men.

[c] Estimated by exponentiation of the coefficient.

[d] See reference [5], pages 194 and 209, 210, for the procedure used to calculate this estimate.

[e] From references.

TC; 7.6 to lower SBP; and 6.1 to nonsmoking—comparable to Cuyler Hammond's "old" estimates of the effects of smoking on life expectancy [24].

While specific data are not given in Table 3, these much more favorable longevity estimates for a cohort with more favorable lifestyles and lifestyle-related major risk factors reflect not only more favorable prognosis in regard to CHD–CVD, but also with respect to several cancers related to smoking and/or diet, and COPD. Again, it must be concluded that the potential for prevention is substantial.

The declines in coronary and cardiovascular mortality in the United States in the last 20–25 years have improved life expectancy for American men and women, black and white, by about 3 years for a person aged 30, 40, or 50. This is with the modest improvements in lifestyles, lifestyle-related risk factors, and medical care achieved until now. The data presented here indicate that with further substantial advances in all these regards, much greater increases in longevity, better health, and better quality of life are achievable.

One can do exactly the same kinds of calculations with Seven Countries Study coefficients [4]. Thus, with use of the data based on 15-year follow-up, with coefficients for the U.S. railroad, northern European, and southern European cohorts for serum TC, SBP, and cigarettes per day (coefficients similar for each of these major risk factors for each of these cohorts, and similar to those for CHA and WE middle-aged men), mean TC of 190 mg/dl compared to 237 mg/dl observed for the U.S. railroad men yields an estimated relative risk of 15-year CHD death of 0.73 (27% lower); SBP of 118 mmHg compared to 135 mmHg observed for the railroad men yields an estimated relative risk of 0.66 (34% lower); no cigarette smoking compared to 10 cigarettes/day (approximate average for the whole railroad cohort) yields an estimated relative risk of 0.73 (27% lower); combined, $0.73 \times 0.66 \times 0.73 = 0.35$, i.e., a relative risk of 15-year CHD death lower by 65% with more favorable status for these three major risk factors compared to the actual levels observed at baseline for the cohort of U.S. railroad men. The situation for the combined northern European cohorts of the Seven Countries Study was similar. Again, the potential for prevention is vast.

All the foregoing data were *estimates* on the potential for prevention with improved lifestyles and consequent lower levels of major risk factors. Until recently, none of the population samples being followed prospectively in the United States or in Europe, including those combined in analyses of the Pooling Project and the Seven Countries Study, were large enough to make possible actual identification of sizeable subcohorts of low-risk men and actual ascertainment of long-term rates of CHD–CVD. Given the adverse lifestyles prevailing throughout "western" populations, middle-aged low-risk men were "rare birds" in these cohorts, few and far between, too few—in prospective studies with samples numbering in the thousands—to make meaningful analysis possible. This became feasible for the first time with long-term follow-up of the remarkable cohort of 361 662 men screened in 1973–1975 in 18 cities across the United States in the recruitment effort of the Multiple Risk Factor Intervention Trial (MRFIT) [8].

Low-risk Men in the MRFIT Cohort. Based on the single set of measurements made in these men, ages 35–57 at baseline, low risk was defined as serum cholesterol under 182 mg/dl (cut point for the lowest quintile), systolic BP < 120 mmHg and diastolic BP < 80 mmHg (clinicians' classic cut points for optimal BP), no current smoking (data on past smoking were not collected), and no history of treatment for diabetes or hospitalization for heart attack. Only 11 098 men (3% of the whole cohort) met these criteria. This finding dots the i's and crosses the t's of the proposition, set down by Geoffrey Rose, that in countries like the United States, because of prevalent lifestyles, populations as a whole are "sick populations" [25]. Therefore, as Henry Blackburn elaborated here, a population-wide, and not just a high-risk, approach is essential to realize the full potential for prevention. Table 4 gives baseline risk-factor data on this MRFIT subcohort, and a second low-risk cohort with serum cholesterol 182–202 mg/dl (second quintile) and all other criteria as described above [26]. These two low-risk subcohorts, singly and combined (11 098 + 9284 = 20 382 men), are compared with the rest of the MRFIT men, exclusive of those with a baseline history of diabetes or heart attack. (Inclusion of men with diabetes or heart attack gives similar results.) For the 11 098 men identified based on the original definition of low risk, mean serum cholesterol was 162 mg/dl, compared to 216 mg/dl for the rest of the cohort, lower by 54 mg/dl; SBP/DBP was 111/72 mmHg, compared to 131/84 mmHg, lower by 20/12 mmHg; mean number of cigarettes per day was, for low-risk men, none versus 10 for the other 322 433 MRFIT men. Table 4 also gives age-adjusted 16-year mortality rates by cause. For the 11 098 low-risk men, compared to the 322 433 men: CHD death rate lower by 86%; stroke, by 78%; all CVD, by 82%. Note also that mortality rates from cancers, other natural causes, and all non-CVD causes were lower for low-risk men, by 40%, 21%, and 30%, respectively. Death rate from violent causes was similar for the two subcohorts—11 098 and 322 433 men. For all-causes mortality, rate for the low-risk subcohort was lower by 52%. Note too that in regard to proportionate mortality, for this low-risk subcohort, CHD—no longer the prime cause of death—accounted for only 9% of all deaths, compared with 31% for the 322 433 men at usual (high) risk.

These much lower long-term mortality rates in the low-risk subcohort (from CHD, stroke, CVD, other natural causes, and all causes) were recorded based on only a one-time measurement of major risk factors, without correction for regression-dilution bias. Therefore, as impressive as are the lower rates for this subcohort, they are still *underestimates* of the potential for prevention. This is the case also for an additional reason: no data were collected in the MRFIT survey of 361 662 men on their patterns of eating, drinking, and exercise. Data on dietary cholesterol-lipid (see above), along with the measurements made, would almost certainly have produced an even finer definition of low risk. For example, it is possible, even likely, that among the two subcohorts of 11 098

Table 4. Baseline risk factor levels and 16-year age-standardized mortality rates by cause, two low-risk strata and other men screened for the Multiple Risk Factor Intervention Trial (MRFIT).

Variable	Low risk Men[b]—serum TC < 182 mg/dl		Low risk Men[b]—serum TC 182–202 mg/dl		Low risk Men—serum TC < 203 mg/dl		All others Men free of DM, MI
Number	11 098		9284		20 382		322 433
Mean serum chol (mg/dl)	162.4		192.1		175.9		216.5
Mean systolic pressure (mmHg)	111.0		111.3		111.2		131.1
Mean diastolic pressure (mmHg)	71.6		72.0		71.8		84.5
Percent smokers	0.0		0.0		0.0		38.7
Mean *n* cigarettes/day, smokers	NA		NA		NA		25.8
Mean age (years)	43.5		44.8		44.1		45.9
16-Year mortality							
Coronary heart disease	39[c]	2.9[d]	76	5.9	115	4.4	10335	21.2
Stroke	5	0.5	11	0.9	16	0.7	1 139	2.3
All CVD	68	5.3	105	8.2	173	6.7	14302	29.4
All non-CVD disease	382	27.3	272	20.4	654	23.8	19069	39.1
Cancers	209	15.4	166	12.8	375	14.1	12546	25.8
Violent causes	73	4.9	46	3.2	119	4.0	2 109	4.4
Other causes[a]	109	7.7	64	4.7	173	6.1	4 717	9.7
All causes	459	33.2	381	28.8	840	30.9	33755	69.3

CVD, cardiovascular diseases; TC, total cholesterol; DM, baseline history of drug treatment for diabetes mellitus; MI baseline history of hospitalization for ≥2 weeks for a heart attack; NA, not applicable.

[a] Other than CVD, cancers, violent causes.

[b] Criteria for low risk at baseline: serum TC < 182 m/dl (quintile 1 of TC distribution), 182–202 mg/dl (quintile 2 of TC distribution), SBP/DBP <120/<80 mmHg; not a smoker; no history of drug treatment for diabetes or hospitalization for 2+ weeks for heart attack.

[c] Number of deaths.

[d] Age standardized death rate per 10000 person-years.

and 9284 men defined as low-risk in Table 4 there were some heavy users of alcohol, who for this reason were not really low-risk.

Given these limitations, the MRFIT data on low risk are all the more remarkable. These actual observations on low risk factor levels at baseline, and their relationship to low 16-year mortality rates, indicate the general validity of estimates of the potential for prevention derived from smaller cohorts. In particular, the data on all-causes death rate, lower by more than 50% for the 11 098 low-risk MRFIT men, also indicate the general validity of estimates that years can be added to life expectancy with health through improvements in lifestyle with prevention and control of major risk factors.

Table 5. Women and men at low risk at baseline and 19-year mortality by cause, Chicago Heart Association Study.

Variable	Women				Men			
	No risk factors[a]		One or more risk factors		No risk factors[a]		One or more risk factors	
Number	231		9881		136		15023	
CHD death	0[b]	0.0[c]	268	14.9	0	0.0	934	35.3
Stroke death	0	0.0	84	4.7	0	0.0	136	5.1
CVD death	0	0.0	402	22.4	0	0.0	1205	45.5
Non-CVD death	9	40.5	700	39.2	4	17.6	1290	48.8
All death	9	40.5	1102	61.6	4	17.6	2495	94.3

CHD, coronary heart disease; CVD, all cardiovascular diseases.
[a] Serum cholesterol < 200 mg/dl, SBP/DBP < 120/< 80 mmHg, never smoked, no diabetes, no history of coronary heart disease (CHD), and no ECG abnormality at baseline; ages 30–69.
[b] Number of deaths.
[c] Age-standardized death rate/10000 person-years.

Low-risk Women and Men in the CHA Cohort. Until 1993, no comparable data were available on women. With 19-year follow-up data now computerized on the Chicago Heart Association Detection Project in Industry (CHA) cohort, analyses on low-risk women as well as men became feasible (Table 5) [27]. For the age group 30–69 years at entry, the cohort of employed women numbered 10112, with 1111 deaths in 19 years, 268 (24.1%) from CHD and 402 (36.2%) from all CVD. Baseline data enable use of six traits to characterize low risk: serum cholesterol under 200 mg/dl, SBP/DBP < 120/< 80 mmHg, never smoked, no diabetes, no history of coronary disease, and no Minnesota Code abnormality on ECG. These latter two were combined as a single criterion. Again, as for the MRFIT cohort, notable is the rarity of low-risk status—only 231 (2.1%) of the women met those criteria. In 19 years of follow-up of these low-risk women, *no* cardiovascular deaths were recorded. Findings were similar for the men: In the total cohort of 15023 men, there were 2499 deaths in 19 years, 934 (37.4%) from CHD and 1205 (48.2%) from all CVD. Only 136 (0.9%) men met all six criteria for low-risk. In this low-risk subcohort, there were *no* CHD or CVD deaths in 19 years and only four non-CVD deaths, so that the age-adjusted mortality rates from non-CVD and all causes were only 36% and 19% of those of all other men. (When those with diabetes, CHD, and/or ECG abnormality at entry were excluded from the comparison, these percentages were 41% and 24%.)

Given the paucity of women and men meeting all six criteria for low risk, further analyses of the CHA data were done, to compare those with any one only or none of the six traits with those having two or more at entry. With current lifestyles in the U.S. population, most of the people had two or more of these traits (Table 6) [27]. Only 1265 (12.5%) of the 10112 women manifested either none or one only of these traits. Their 19-year coronary

Table 6. Women and men with none or one only of six risk factors[a] at baseline and 19-year mortality by cause, Chicago Heart Association Study.

Variable	Women				Men			
	No or 1 risk factor only		2+ risk factors		No or 1 risk factor only		2+ risk factors	
Number	1265		8847		984		14175	
CHD Death	2[b]	1.2[c]	266	15.8	8	6.7	926	36.5
Stroke Death	3	2.3	81	4.9	4	4.3	132	5.2
CVD Death	7	5.2	395	23.6	15	12.8	1190	46.9
Non-CVD Death	47	29.2	662	40.3	42	31.9	1252	49.5
All Death	54	34.4	1057	63.9	57	44.7	2442	96.3

CHD, coronary heart diseases; CVD, all cardiovascular diseases.
[a] Serum total cholesterol <200 mg/dl, SBP/DBP <120/<80 mmHg, never smoked, no diabetes, no history of coronary heart disease, no ECG abnormality at baseline; ages 30–69.
[b] Number of deaths.
[c] Age-standardized death rate/10000 person-years.

mortality was lower by 92% compared to the rate among the remaining women, all CVD mortality was lower by 78%, non-CVD mortality was lower by 28%, and all-causes mortality was lower by 46%. The corresponding analysis for men yielded similar results: only 984 (6.5%) of the 15175 men manifested none or one only of the six traits; for these 984 men, 19-year age-adjusted death rates were much lower than for the 14175 men with two or more of the six traits— mortality rates lower by 82% for CHD, by 73% for CVD, by 36% for non-CVD, and by 54% for all-causes mortality. Again, these are underestimates of the potential for prevention, both because of regression-dilution bias (one measurement per person of the six traits) and because no data were collected on other important risk factors such as eating, drinking, and exercise habits.

Dietary Factors Influencing Serum Cholesterol and Blood Pressure

All of this is well and good, but can one really prevent and control these adverse traits to a significant degree?

Dietary Influences on Serum Cholesterol. Medical journals even today publish reports that blood cholesterol cannot be much influenced. Everyone here is aware that as long ago as the 1960s, Keys, Grande, and Anderson showed, in metabolic ward experiments, that dietary lipid composition, dietary fiber, and calorie balance all influence serum cholesterol levels [28–33]. These classic studies, and those of many other research groups, demonstrate unequivocally that *large* reductions in serum cholesterol occur with substantial improvements in eating patterns. The massive data on dietary lipid effects were reviewed earlier this year by Mark Hegsted and colleagues [34], who also did invaluable research in this area. Recently Keys and Hegsted jointly received a prestigious award for these research contributions.

Quantitative estimates merit citation. The two similar regression equations on the relationship of isocaloric change in dietary lipids to change in serum cholesterol, derived by Keys et al. and by Hegsted et al. from scores of metabolic ward type experiments, are

$$\text{A.} \quad \Delta TC = 1.35(2\Delta S - \Delta P) + 1.5\sqrt{\Delta C} \; [28\text{--}31]$$

$$\text{B.} \quad \Delta TC = 2.10\Delta S - 1.16\Delta P + 0.067\Delta C \; [34]$$

where Δ is change and S and P are percent total kilocalories from dietary saturates and polyunsaturates and C is dietary cholesterol in milligrams per 1000 kilocalories.

For U.S. adults, a halving of dietary saturates and cholesterol from current average levels of about 14% of kilocalories and 160 mg/1000 Kcal, respectively, can be predicted to yield a serum TC fall of about 22 mg/dl (from equation A, 23.5 mg/dl; from equation B, 20.1 mg/dl; mean of the two, 21.8 mg/dl). With mean serum cholesterol of U.S. adults averaging about 205 mg/dl [35], this is a fall of almost 11%. Add to this the effect of a modest increase in dietary polyunsaturates, from 6% of kilocalories to 9%, producing a further fall in serum TC of almost 4 mg/dl, and the total decrease is about 26 mg/dl, almost 13%.

Repeated assessments indicate the applicability of these predictions to the general population (e.g., see the detailed analyses of the National Diet–Heart Study [36]). With a 1% serum TC fall estimated to lower CHD risk of middle-aged men by 2%, these changes predict a 26% reduction in CHD, without any consideration of the independent effect of dietary lipid-cholesterol on risk (see above). For young adult men, the predicted effect on long-term CHD risk is far greater: A 1% decrease in serum TC yields a 5% reduction in CHD risk (again, see above). Finally, since repeated assertions have been made that the effect of dietary cholesterol on TC is negligible, it is important to emphasize that in the above predictions, about one-fifth of the TC reduction is due to the halving of dietary cholesterol intake. Again, it is relevant also to note the further potential benefit from this particular dietary improvement, given the multiple data sets (see above) indicating an independent effect of diet cholesterol on CHD risk, over and above its adverse influence on serum TC and its possible adverse effect on blood pressure (see below).

Additive favorable effects on serum TC and its fractions are obtained when dietary lipid modifications along the foregoing lines are combined with in-creased intake of water-soluble fibers from legumes, other vegetables, fruits, and oat products. For example, in a recent Canadian study of hyperlipidemic men and women, with dietary fat modification plus increased ingestion of about 6 g/day of such fiber, decrease in serum cholesterol was greater by

16 mg/dl than with fat modification alone—a reduction of 13.9% *vs* 8.0% (from a baseline mean level of 265 mg/dl) [37]. Similar results were obtained in a study of hyperlipidemic monks in The Netherlands [38]. Detailed assessment has not been made of the quantitative influences of water-soluble dietary fibers on serum cholesterol, in contrast to the regression analyses measuring the effects of dietary lipid change on serum cholesterol [28–31,34]. From a survey of recent reports, including three studies of oat products by our group [39–41], it seems that adults with hypercholesterolemia (e.g., ≥200 mg/dl) are more responsive to water-soluble fibers than those with TC under 200 mg/dl, a phenomenon that prevails also in regard to responsiveness to dietary lipid modification [28–31,36]. As a first approximation, a reasonable estimate is that for those with TC ≥ 200 mg/dl (group mean of about 240–260 mg/dl), each additional ingested gram of water-soluble fiber produces about a 3.0 mg/dl fall in TC, that is, a fall of more than 1% over and above that resulting from dietary fat modification. From U.S. experience, for the adult population overall, with mean serum cholesterol nowadays of about 205 mg/dl, each additional ingested gram of water-soluble fiber leads to a TC fall of about 1 to 2 mg/dl (0.5% to 1.0%) over and above effects of dietary lipid modification.

Available data indicate that water-soluble fiber ingestion averages about 4 g/day for American adults, with a variation across quintiles of this distribution ranging from about 1 to 9 g/day (MRFIT nutrition monograph, submission pending, 1994). It is therefore realistic to project a first goal of doubling the average intake, to a level of 8 g/day, in accordance with national recommendations for increased vegetable and fruit intake to help prevent several major chronic diseases [42]. The result would be an estimated enhancement of serum TC reduction by 2% to 4%. Again keep in mind the estimate: A 1% TC fall yields a 2% CHD decrease. A second goal is to increase average water-soluble fiber intake to 12 g/day.

For overweight people, moderate weight loss on a fat-modified diet also yields additive favorable influence on TC and all its fractions. This was shown in the 1960s in the National Diet–Heart Study [36]. It was the finding both for free-living participants and for institutionalized men in Minnesota. The data on the latter are particularly meaningful since dietary lipid composition was thoroughly controlled and known. For men fed diet B, reduced in total fat, saturates, and cholesterol, and moderately increased in poly fat, in the absence of weight loss, serum cholesterol fell 14.1%, whereas for those experiencing moderate weight loss (about 4% on average, 2.7 kg) serum cholesterol fell 19.4%, that is, a decline greater by about 38%. MRFIT has similar findings (MRFIT nutrition monograph, submission pending, 1994).

The estimated combined impact on population mean serum cholesterol of all three nutritional improvements is: dietary fat modification (ΔS: from 14% of kilocalories to 7%; ΔC: from 160 to 80 mg/1000 Kcal; ΔP: from 6% of kilocalories to 9%) yields a 26 mg/dl TC fall. Reduction in body mass index from an average level of about 26 to 24 kg/m^2 gives an additional decline in TC of 10 mg/dl. The combined effect of fat modification and weight control is estimated to be 36 mg/dl. Increase in water-soluble fiber intake by 4 g/day gives an additional decline in TC of about 6 mg/dl. Thus, total TC fall is estimated as 42 mg/dl. Based on the NHANES-III latest data for mean TC level for U.S. adults of about 205 mg/dl [36], this estimated decline would be to a mean level of 163 mg/dl, similar to adult mean levels in Japan and China, and constituting a fall of 20.5%.

Is such a low population mean serum cholesterol level a realistic projection for "western" populations? In my judgment, yes. By way of support, I remind you first of the decline in mean levels already recorded by American adults, from about 235 mg/dl in the 1950s to about 220 in the early 1960s to 205 in the late 1980s and early 1990s, an overall decrease so far of about 13% [35,43]. Second, recall the values recorded in the Boston commune study of young adults eating a macrobiotic diet, compared to findings for Framingham young adults: mean TC of 126 mg/dl for the former, 184 mg/dl for the latter, a difference of 58 mg/dl (31.5%) [44]. Third, recall the median values for the two Japanese cohorts in the Seven Countries Study of about 160 to 170 mg/dl [45,46]; the similar levels for middle-aged men employed by the Japan National Railways [47]; the mean level of 181 mg/dl for middle-aged Japanese men in the Ni-Hon-San Study [48]; and the even lower mean levels of about 155 mg/dl for southern rural Chinese men and women studied as recently as 1983–1984 [49]. These lower mean levels for East Asian populations reflect differences in lifestyles, particularly in eating patterns and consequent nutrient composition (also in regard to calorie balance and habitual physical activity). They show what the "human condition" can be for this important prognostic variable, serum cholesterol, given more favorable lifestyles. Once again, the potential for prevention is *great*.

Dietary Influences on Blood Pressure. Little has been said here about factors influencing blood pressure, one of the mines that merits extensive digging in the Seven Countries Study data.

Conceived in Finland in 1982, at the First Advanced Ten-Day International Teaching Seminar on Cardiovascular Epidemiology and Prevention, the international cooperative INTERSALT Study has accrued valuable data, both cross-population and within-population, on relationships of dietary factors to BP. This study was done with high-level standardization [50] based on a common protocol and five regional training sessions for staff, who surveyed 52 population samples from 32 countries—three in Japan, one in Korea, two in India, three in the People's Republic of China, one in Taiwan, and the others in Europe, North and South America, Africa, and the south Pacific, including four isolated preliterate populations (Yanomamo and Xingu Indians in Brazil, highlanders of Papua New Guinea, and a rural sample in Kenya in lifestyle transition) [51]. At each local center, the effort was made to recruit 200 men and women ages 20–59.

One important ecologic finding was that sample median 24-h sodium (Na) excretion related significantly and independently to slope of systolic pressure

Fig. 2. INTERSALT Study cross-population (ecologic) analysis on relationship between population sample-adjusted median 24-h sodium excretion and sample-adjusted linear slope of systolic blood pressure with age (age 20 to 59), all 52 samples; adjustments were for age, sex, body mass index, and alcohol intake. (Data from [51])

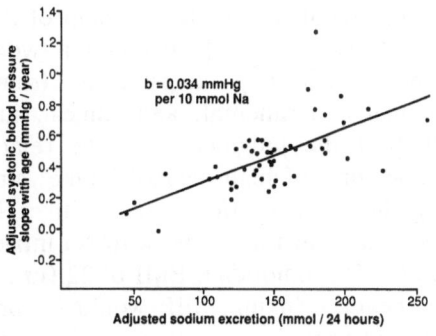

Table 7. Relationship for individuals of 24-h urinary sodium and potassium excretion, body mass index, and heavy alcohol use to systolic blood pressure in 10 079 men and women ages 20–59, INTERSALT Study.

Variable	Coefficient[a]	Difference	SBP difference (mmHg)
Na	0.0313[b]	170–70	−3.1
K	−0.0671[b]	55–90	−2.3
BMI	0.733[c]	25–22	−2.2
Alcohol	3.544[d]	14%–0%	−0.5

[a] Multivariate adjusted for reliability [59,60].
[b] mmHg per mmol Na, K.
[c] mmHg per unit BMI.
[d] mmHg, heavy alcohol use (≥300 ml/week) vs no alcohol use.

with age (Fig. 2) [51]. The coefficient from the multiple linear regression analysis was 0.034 mmHg/mmol Na per year. That is, for a population sample with median 24-h Na excretion lower by 100 mmol Na (e.g., 70 *vs* 170 mmol), SBP slope over 30 years (e.g., age 25 to age 55) was on average about 10 mmHg smaller (e.g., upward slope 4 *vs* 14 mmHg) [18,51–55]. A similar relation was seen between median sample Na and slope diastolic BP with age.

In its within-population analyses, dealing with the 10 079 individual INTERSALT participants, the study recorded significant findings on the independent relation of 24-h sodium excretion, BMI, and heavy alcohol intake to systolic pressure (Table 7) [18,51–57]. In multiple linear regression analyses, each was positively related to SBP, with control for the other two as well as for age and sex and for 24-h urinary potassium, calcium, and magnesium excretion. Further, in these multivariate analyses, there was a significant independent inverse relationship of 24-h urinary potassium excretion to SBP (Table 7) [18,51–57]. As noted in two recent public policy statements and elsewhere [18,58–60], extensive data from studies of many types—epidemiologic, animal experimental, and clinical, including randomized controlled trials—support the judgment that the relationships of dietary intake of salt and potassium, of high alcohol intake, and of body mass to BP are etiologically significant. The effects are additive. Thus, the INTERSALT data led to the estimate that for people with Na intake of 70 (vs 170) mmol/day, K intake of 90 (vs 55) mmol/day, BMI of 22 (vs 25) kg/m², and zero (vs 14%) prevalence of heavy drinking, SBP would be on average 8.1 mmHg lower. Data from clinical trials indicate that smaller improvements in these four traits result in control and prevention of high blood pressure in a significant proportion of hypertensive or hypertension-prone adults [59–63]. Moreover, on a population-wide basis, community intervention to lower salt intake was shown to be effective in reducing SBP and DBP in a trial in Portugal, a country with one of the highest levels of per capita salt ingestion and rates of high BP [64].

From multiple data sets on the relationship of SBP to incidence and mortality from CHD, stroke, and all CVD as well as to all-causes mortality, it is estimated that a shift downward of the SBP distribution of 8.1 mmHg on average would result in considerable impact on disease rates. Thus, for young adult men, based on CHA long-term data, death rates would be lower by 13% for CHD, 17% for CVD, and 9% for all causes. For middle-aged men, based on data from the Western Electric, MRFIT, CHA, and Seven Countries Studies, long-term CHD death rate would be lower by 9% (CHA) to 35% (southern European, Seven Countries), CVD death rate by 9% (CHA) to 17% (MRFIT), and all-causes death rate by 7% (CHA) to 12% (MRFIT, WE). For older men, from CHA data, death rate would be lower by 7% from CHD and CVD, and 5% from all causes. For middle-aged women, from CHA data, death rate would be lower by 12% from CHD, 13% from CVD, and 7% from all causes. For older women, from CHA data, death rate would be lower by 13% from CHD and CVD and by 10% from all causes. For a country like the United States, savings in lives lost per year would number in the tens of thousands [18,54,55]. Since the slope of the relationship of BP to risk of stroke is even steeper than to risk of CHD [15], this 8.1-mmHg shift downward of the SBP distribution would have even greater effects on incidence and mortality from stroke [18,54,55].

Although the INTERSALT coefficients in Table 7 are multivariate adjusted for regression-dilution bias, for other reasons it is likely that those for Na and K particularly are underestimates. These reasons were presented in detail to the Third International Conference on Nutrition in Cardio-Cerebrovascular Diseases held in 1992 in Aomori, northern Japan, and are published [18]. For example, a comprehensive review of cross-population, within-population, and intervention studies on salt and BP produced the estimate that ingestion of a diet lower in sodium by 100 mmol/day leads on average to SBP lower by

5 mmHg (cf. Table 7), and the effects are even greater for older people and for those with higher SBP [63].

One other set of INTERSALT findings merits emphasis: For individuals in many of its 52 population samples, an inverse association was found between educational attainment and blood pressure. A significant proportion of the higher BP levels in INTERSALT participants with less education was accounted for by their higher levels of BMI, Na and alcohol intake, and lower levels of K intake [65]. These are the first data showing that, as long suspected, less favorable lifestyle patterns related to less education play a role in the inverse association between education and BP. Strata of lower socioeconomic status in several industrialized countries (including the United States) not only have more adverse patterns of BP, but also of serum cholesterol, body mass, diabetes, cigarette use, CHD–CVD–all-causes mortality, and trends of mortality (see below). Therefore, these INTERSALT findings have important implications in relation to challenges confronting medical care and public health efforts to realize the potential for prevention equally in all SES strata of the population.

At present, in the second major phase of its research, INTERSALT is assessing relationships to BP of markers of protein intake in 24-h urine, including total nitrogen and urea N, and sulphate as an indicator of ingested S-containing amino acids. Total N in 24-h urine has been termed a "gold standard" for assessment of total protein intake, as Professor Fidanza has noted here. Urea N accounts for most total N, and the two are very highly correlated in rank order analyses. Most of the sulphate in urine is derived from ingested S-containing amino acids (cystine, cysteine, methionine). Biochemical analyses on 24-h urine samples from the 10 079 participants are in progress at the INTERSALT Central Laboratory, University of Leuven, Belgium, under the direction of Professor Hugo Kesteloot. As reported to national and international scientific meetings [66,67], data for almost half the participants, from 26 of the 52 samples worldwide, show significant *inverse* relationships between each of these three markers of protein intake and BP (both SBP and DBP), with control for age, sex, BMI, alcohol intake, and 24-h urinary excretions of Na, K, Ca, and Mg. The magnitude of the pooled regression coefficients (even without adjustment for regression-dilution bias) indicates that these relationships—if verified in the final analyses for all 10 079 participants and by other studies—could be of practical importance. It is particularly relevant therefore to note here that Japanese colleagues, based on their research in human populations and animals, have called attention to the possibility that intake of protein, and particularly of certain amino acids (among them S-containing amino acids) seems to have favorable effects on BP [68,69], contrary to the opposite opinion generally prevailing among researchers in "western" countries. Chinese colleagues also have presented evidence from both cross-population and within-population observational studies indicating an inverse relationship between dietary protein and BP [70,71].

Stimulated by these INTERSALT findings, this matter has been under exploration with use of several other data sets: on men randomized into MRFIT [72]; on men in the Western Electric Study [73]; on the CARDIA samples of black and white young adult men and women in the United States [74]; on women in the Nurses Health Study and men in the study of health professionals in the United States (F. Sacks, personal communication); on male and female participants in a recent U.K. national nutrition survey [75]. Results have been generally concordant with the INTERSALT findings in regard to an independent inverse association between protein intake and BP. It remains to be clarified whether total protein intake is critically important, or whether differential effects prevail for protein from specific sources (e.g., animal, vegetable) or for specific amino acids.

The MRFIT analyses, based on four or five 24-h dietary recalls during 6 years of participation by each of 12000+ men randomized into the trial, explored relationships of multiple dietary factors to SBP and DBP (also measured annually during the 6 years). Even with four or five recalls per man, the estimate was that for most of the dietary factors observed, regression coefficients would be no more than about 50% of true coefficients; considerable regression-dilution bias would remain, albeit much less than with use of only one 24-h recall [18,19]. In accordance with INTERSALT findings, in multiple linear regression analyses of the MRFIT data there were significant independent direct relationships of BMI, alcohol use, and Na intake (or dietary Na/K) to SBP and DBP with control for age, race, education, smoking at baseline and during the trial, and serum cholesterol [72]. There was also a significant independent inverse relationship of dietary K to SBP and DBP, and—as mentioned above—of dietary protein to BP (specifically, DBP). Among other macronutrients, significant independent direct relationships were recorded with DBP for dietary cholesterol, saturates, hence for Keys score as well. While the effect of each macronutrient was apparently modest without correction for regression-dilution bias, it became greater with multivariate correction for this problem, and the estimated combined effects on SBP and DBP were considerable. Thus, these data underscore the possibilities for marked improvements in population BP means and distributions through improved nutrition. This being the case, it is urgent that additional research efforts be mounted to test the reproducibility of these new findings on dietary macronutrients and BP. Such studies must be able to deal satisfactorily with the now clearly identified methodological problems. This is a prerequisite for resolving uncertainties concerning these important issues of the influence of multiple dietary factors on BP. The two key methodologic issues are: the essentiality of large sample sizes for power to detect small effects on BP of each dietary factor, and the essentiality of high-quality methods to assess usual dietary intake of individuals, to overcome the problem of high ratio of intra- to interindividual variability for dietary factors [19]. With "cheap and dirty" methods (small sample sizes, only one 24-h recall per person or a short food frequency questionnaire), false-negative results are built in. A mix of "findings" of direct, inverse, or no relationships gives total confusion, a "penny-wise and pound-foolish" situation in the long run. Ancel Keys wrote clearly about this problem years ago [16]. It has taken a long time for the lesson to get learned—and this is still pending in all too many quarters [19].

Of the cited investigations on dietary factors influencing BP, the Western Electric Study is unusual in having in-depth repeat high-quality data on baseline dietary patterns of its participants (see above), followed by annual examinations with BP measurement for 9 years. These data make possible not only cross-sectional but also prospective analyses on relationships of multiple baseline dietary factors to evolution of SBP and DBP over years. At the March 1993 scientific sessions of the Council on Epidemiology and Prevention of the American Heart Association, my colleague Professor Kiang Liu presented such Western Electric data, using the Generalized Estimating Equation (GEE) computer program to assess both cross-sectional and prospective relationships [73]. The prospective analyses yielded data on associations of baseline dietary variables both to average SBP and DBP during the next 9 years and to annual change in BP. At baseline, as expected, significant independent direct relationships were found for age, BMI, alcohol intake, and SBP, and education was inversely related to SBP. All these variables also related significantly and independently to average SBP during the 9 years of follow-up. (No data were available on dietary Na and K intake.) Change in BMI during follow-up related significantly and directly to serial change in SBP—BMI higher by $1 \, kg/m^2$ (about 3 kg) was associated with annual SBP increase greater by 1.7 mmHg. Although macronutrients were not significantly related to BP at baseline, prospective analyses showed direct relationships of dietary cholesterol ($P < 0.01$), S ($P < 0.10 > 0.05$), and Keys score ($P < 0.01$) to annual change in SBP during the 9-year follow-up and inverse relationships of vegetable protein and total carbohydrate to SBP change ($P < 0.05$), with control in each of these separate analyses for baseline BMI, alcohol intake, cigarettes per day, education, and age. For example, Keys score of 60 was associated with annual SBP increase of 1.6 mmHg, compared to an increase of 1.1 mmHg/year with a score of 30. Thus, over 9 years of follow-up, lower intake of cholesterol and saturates plus higher intake of polyunsaturates, yielding a Keys score lower by 30, gives an estimated smaller rise in SBP of 4.5 mmHg.

In further analyses carried out subsequent to this cited presentation, relationships have been explored of baseline vitamin C and beta-carotene intake to annual change in BP during the 9 years of post-baseline follow-up of the Western Electric men. In separate analyses, both with and without inclusion of Keys score among the multiple variables assessed, there was a significant inverse relationship of each of these antioxidant vitamins to change in SBP (Table 8) [76]. For the two variables considered in this table, more favorable intake (the vitamin in the upper quartile, Keys score in the lower quartile) was associated with a combined effect estimated to be 2.8 to 3.0 mmHg over 10 years of follow-up.

Table 8. Baseline dietary vitamin C, beta-carotene, Keys score, and average annual systolic blood pressure change, 1958–1966, Western Electric Study[a].

Variable	Coefficient (Z score) (mmHg/yr/unit nutrient)	75th% vs 25th% 10-year effect (mmHg)
Vitamin C (mg/day)[b]	−0.0028 (−2.41)	−1.4
Keys score[c]	+0.0157 (+2.55)	+1.6
Beta-carotene (IU/day)[d]	−0.000041 (−2.42)	−1.2
Keys score	+0.0157 (+2.48)	+1.6

[a] 1802 men ages 40–55 at baseline; analyses controlled for age, kilocalories per day, body mass index, education, alcohol per day, cigarettes per day, other nutrients.
[b] Vitamin C—75th% 40.5 mg/1000 Kcal; 25th% 23.8 mg/1000 Kcal.
[c] Keys score—$1.35 (2S - P) + 1.5\sqrt{C}$, where S is % kcal from saturated fats, P is % kcal from polyunsaturated fats, and C is dietary cholesterol in mg/1000 Kcal [28–31].
[d] Beta-carotene, 75th% 2245 and 25th% 1286 IU/1000 Kcal.

Thus, for each of the macro- and micronutrients assessed in these prospective Western Electric analyses, the data indicate quantitative effects that have potential practical importance for the improvement of population BP distributions and their change over time, *if* further research confirms these findings, leading to the judgment that the relationships are etiologically significant. These are nutritional effects on BP and change in BP independent of BMI and alcohol intake. Their independence from dietary Na and K intake (also Mg, fiber) remains to be determined. Clearly, once again a high-quality multifaceted research assault to answer these important questions merits highest priority, for both practical and theoretical reasons [19]. In the interim, current recommendations for optimal nutrition—in regard to calorie balance, alcohol, Na, K, dietary lipids, and dietary sources (fruits, vegetables) of antioxidant and other micronutrients [42]—merit widespread currency for many reasons, including beneficial effects on BP. Here too, as well as in regard to population serum cholesterol-lipid levels, the potential is great for prevention of increased levels with age and for achievement of much more favorable adult means and distributions, with consequent important preventive impact on CHD, stroke, CVD, all-causes mortality, and longevity.

In several countries (including both Japan and the United States), CHD, stroke, CVD, and hence all-causes death rates have declined considerably (Figs. 1, 3, 4). A part of this achievement almost certainly relates to blood pressure reductions achieved both by improved lifestyles and by pharmacologic means. Much more can be achieved through safe, optimal nutrition, beginning early in life, for the primary prevention of adverse distributions of both blood pressure and serum cholesterol in all strata of the population.

But—it is argued—all said above on the potential impact on disease is based on estimation or inference. What about "direct evidence," as in data from

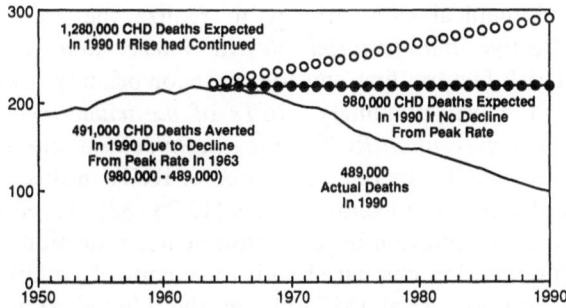

Fig. 3. Trend of age-adjusted mortality rate (per 100 000 population) (*solid line*) from coronary heart disease (CHD), 1950–1990, United States, all persons. Expected numbers of CHD deaths in 1990 if the rise in rate from 1950 to 1963 had continued (*open circles*), or if the peak rate of 1963 had persisted (*solid circles*). Observed number of CHD deaths, 1990. (Data from [77])

Fig. 4. Trends of age-standardized mortality rates (per 100 000 population) from cerebrovascular disease (stroke) and ischemic heart disease (IHD), Japan, 1950 to 1989, men and women ages 40–69 years. (Data from [2])

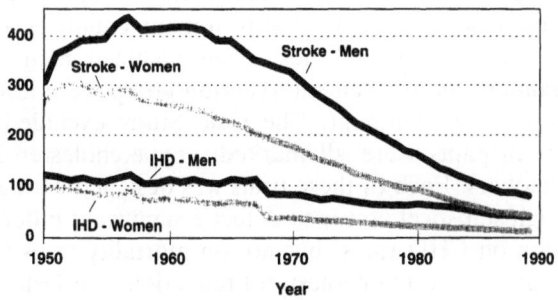

randomized controlled trials (RCTs) with "hard" disease end points (clinical, angiographic)? A review of RCTs is beyond the scope of this report. However, it may be useful to deal with two key aspects, since there seems to be confusion among some colleagues about the import of data from RCTs, particularly on serum cholesterol reduction.

The Multifactorial RCTs. My first concern is with the importance of results from RCTs using multifactorial intervention to control combinations of major risk factors. As emphasized above, the four major risk factors—unbalanced dietary pattern, diet-dependent adverse distributions of serum cholesterol and blood pressure, and cigarette smoking—have *multiplicative* effects on CHD–CVD risk. Thus, combinations of these traits have especially deleterious effects. Such combinations are widely prevalent in the adult populations age 30+ of many industrialized countries. As the other side of the coin, presence of *none* of them or any one only, is generally rare in adult populations, and predicts low CHD–CVD risk. From these key facts it follows that the cornerstone of public health and medical care strategy to realize the great potential for prevention is effective *multifactorial lifestyle intervention*, to prevent and control all major risk factors, first and foremost for primary prevention in the general population. Correspondingly, *RCTs of particular meaning and consequence are primary prevention RCTs testing multifactorial intervention against these major risk factors*. But among the scores of RCTs in this field, only four were multifactorial primary prevention trials [12,78–83]. Three of these were generally successful in achieving at least modest net reductions in major risk factors in their intervention compared with their control groups: the Multiple Risk Factor Intervention Trial (MRFIT) in the United States, the World Health Organization Collaborative Trial in Europe, and the Oslo Study in Norway [78–82]. All three focused on assessing ability to achieve primary prevention in middle-aged men. Each involved counseling of their intervention group to achieve smoking cessation and improved eating patterns, particularly in regard to dietary lipids, to lower serum cholesterol. Nutritional recommendations included reductions in total fat, saturated fat, and dietary cholesterol, along with modest increase in polyunsaturates. Thus they were trials—*the only such*—involving the dietary patterns repeatedly advocated for the general population by expert groups in many countries and by WHO [12,42,84–88].

The first two of these trials included men with high BP, and such men randomized to their intervention group were also candidates for antihypertensive drug treatment. The Oslo Study excluded men with high BP; its 1232 participants were all markedly hypercholesterolemic, and almost 80% were smokers. Each of these trials was designed with a sample size estimated to give high statistical power to detect a significant influence of multifactorial intervention on CHD rates, but not on mortality rates from all causes. Particularly in regard to serum cholesterol reduction, the Oslo Study was the most successful of the three in achieving a sustained net fall in serum cholesterol—10% (intervention group minus control group) throughout the several years of the trial, compared to a net decrease of about 3% for the other two trials. As spelled out in greater detail in a recent editorial [12], each of these three trials recorded favorable results not only for CHD (incidence, mortality), but also (with long-term follow-up) for death from all causes. Percentage-wise, the Oslo Study reductions in end-point rates were the greatest. At the end of the planned 5 years of intervention, incidence of first major CHD events was 47% lower in the intervention than in the control group ($P = 0.028$, two-tailed test); CHD mortality was 56% lower ($P = 0.086$); all-causes mortality was 31% lower ($P = 0.246$) [81]. At 15-year follow-up, CHD mortality was 48% lower in the intervention than in the control group ($P = 0.006$, two-tailed test) and all-causes mortality was 26% lower ($P = 0.056$, two-tailed test) [82]. None of these three trials had excess non-CVD mortality (cancer, violence, other) in its intervention group. The favorable findings of these three multifactorial trials are concordant with the data from long-term epidemiologic studies indicating the potential for prevention of CHD–CVD incidence, and all-causes mortality as well, through control of the major risk factors. They are also concordant with the population-wide experience of many countries, including Japan and the United States (see Figs. 1, 3, 4), that have registered progress in recent decades in public health and medical care efforts to improve lifestyles and control the major CVD risk factors. In these countries, substantial declines have occurred not only in CHD, stroke, and CVD mortality, but also in all-causes mortality.

Meta-analyses of Unifactorial RCTs on Serum Cholesterol Reduction. Despite the above cited array of evidence, as well as multiple other supportive data sets from clinical investigation and animal experimentation, in recent years a few authors of meta-analyses of RCTs have alleged that serum cholesterol reduction is harmful, especially when used for CHD primary prevention, that is, results in excess mortality from non-CHD, non-CVD, and all causes [12,89–91]. An assumption (unstated) underlies these meta-analyses, which uncritically combine data from RCTs with diverse interventions (several drugs, surgery, high polyunsaturated fat diets). This assumption is that only their influence on serum cholesterol counts, and nothing else about their effects matters; hence they all can be included in a single meta-analysis. For example, one report combined data from 26 RCTs, 17 of them involving intervention with seven different drugs (cholestyramine, clofibrate, colestipol, dextrothyroxine, estrogens, gemfibrizol, and nicotinic acid) [90], including the five medication regimens in the Coronary Drug Project (CDP). But for three of the CDP groups, active drug was stopped early due to adverse effects, compared to placebo, without countervailing favorable findings (dextrothyroxine, 2.5 mg estrogen, 5.0 mg estrogen) [92–97]. In contrast, CDP results were significantly favorable for its nicotinic acid group compared to placebo [96,97]. Combining such opposite findings in a meta-analysis results in concealing important differences in outcome among drug regimens. I have been involved in the CDP since its beginning in the 1960s, as chair of its steering committee. At no time in the years of work of this national cooperative group, including skilled clinicians, epidemiologists, statisticians, and others, was it ever considered appropriate to combine outcome data from the five separate active treatment groups for comparison with the placebo group. It was explicitly understood that the CDP active treatment groups were receiving medications of different types, pharmacology, mechanisms of action, side effects, possible toxic effects, and so on. Hence *each had to be tested separately—as provided by the CDP design—for efficacy in secondary prevention.* Meta-analyses combining such different treatments are fatally flawed. Conclusions based on such meta-analyses are without scientific foundation, are erroneous in regard to the etiologic relationship of the major risk factors to CHD–CVD and in regard to the potential for prevention, and are irrelevant for public policy.

National Public Policy and Its Effective Implementation to Realize the Potential for Prevention

A scientific foundation is a necessary but not a sufficient prerequisite for a successful public health and medical care effort in the population to realize the potential for prevention [1]. In addition, proper *national public policy* is essential, dedicated to achieving that potential across the entire population of both sexes, all ages, geographic areas, ethnic groups, socioeconomic levels, and cultural backgrounds. This dedicated public policy in turn requires sustained allocation of adequate resources for its implementation. This is the lesson of successes—and failures—in the control of past epidemics (e.g., diphtheria, tuberculosis, pellagra) and contemporary ones (e.g., CHD in "western" industrialized countries, stroke in Japan, AIDS worldwide) [98–100].

Development of National Public Policy on CHD–Stroke–CVD Prevention

The United States was one of the first—if not the first—country to develop such a public policy. Here at this meeting celebrating 35 years of the Seven Countries Study and Ancel Keys' 90th birthday, it is especially appropriate to call attention to the first document addressed to the public on the possibility of prevention through improved lifestyles—the 1959 *Statement on Arteriosclerosis* sponsored by Professor Keys' colleague and friend, colleague and friend of many of us, Dr. Paul Dudley White, along with a group of senior cardiologists and CVD researchers [101]. In that same year the American Heart Association issued its first statement on smoking and CVD health, two years later its landmark diet statement [84], and a few years thereafter its general statement on risk factors, all reiterated and reinforced in updated form right down to the present [86,102,103]. In 1964 came the historic *Report to the Surgeon General on Smoking and Health* [104], the first federal government policy commitment. This was followed in subsequent years by the Report of the White House Conference on Nutrition; the Dietary Guidelines from the U.S. Senate Select Committee on Nutrition and Human Needs; the Report on the Primary Prevention of the Atherosclerotic Diseases from the Inter-Society Commission on Heart Disease Resources [85]; the launching of the National High Blood Pressure Education Program (NHBEP) [58,59], under the aegis of the National Heart, Lung, and Blood Institute (NHLBI), so that by the 1970s, elements of a national governmental policy commitment were in place. This federal commitment was further strengthened and extended in important ways in the 1980s and 1990s [12,59,105–113]. A most recent and very important development is the commitment by the NHBEP–NHLBI to a national policy for the *primary prevention of high blood pressure* by nutritional-hygienic means, the first such national initiative in any country [59].

These years-long developments of U.S. government policy for CHD–CVD prevention took place, deliberately, with broad support from more than a score of major national organizations of physicians and other health professionals, and from the American Heart Association (AHA). Throughout, AHA has played a major and decisive role. It is a reasonable judgment that its endeavors for coronary prevention in the United States, including positively influencing U.S. governmental policy, account decisively for the pace-setting nature internationally of U.S. lifestyle improvements, risk-factor reductions, and declines in CHD–CVD mortality rates. Organizations like AHA—large national voluntary health agencies—seem to be uniquely American, combining large numbers of health professionals and concerned citizens from the general public in their membership, leadership, and multifaceted activities, with a grass-roots structure reaching into about every community in the country.

During the 1960s and 1970s, several other countries experiencing the coronary epidemic also developed national policy positions aimed at its control. These related particularly to population patterns of dietary lipid intake and cigarette use (e.g., in Scandinavian countries, Finland, Australia). Ancel Keys contributed to the development of the dietary recommendations, in Europe and the United States as well [87]. In Japan, efforts were initiated for reduction of the high incidence and mortality rates from stroke, the major form of CVD in Far Eastern countries. These included recommendations for reduction of the high salt intake prevailing in the population, and for the detection, evaluation, and sustained pharmacologic treatment of the large numbers of people with high blood pressure, the most important risk factor for strokes of every type.

In 1982, the World Health Organization published its *Expert Committee Report on the Prevention of Coronary Heart Disease* [88]. This has had wide circulation and great influence. Our good colleague and friend, Geoffrey Rose (recently deceased), was chair of this Expert Committee, and Henry Blackburn was its rapporteur. Deliberately, thanks to Professor Rose's profound thinking, this Report for the first time presented in fully developed form the basic concept of a *population-wide preventive approach*, as well as a high-risk approach, as essential for control of the CHD epidemic. This idea had previously been embodied in policy recommendations on nutrition, as those of the American Heart Association and later the U.S. government, but its meaning and importance had not been explicitly elaborated. Professor Rose grasped intellectually the relevance of so doing, and took pains to make this the central conceptual thrust of the WHO Report. Shortly after his retirement, he wrote in depth on this important theme in a monograph [114]. All of us are deeply in his debt for this invaluable contribution.

Implementation of National Public Policy on CHD–Stroke–CVD Prevention

In the United States and other countries throughout these decades, resources allocated to implement policies for CHD–stroke–CVD prevention have been modest. This is the case for governmental budgetary appropriations (national, regional, state, county, local) and for expenditures by voluntary and private organizations, including the American Heart Association. This fact is readily demonstrated by several statistics: the percentage spent on CHD–CVD prevention in national health budgets; dollars spent per capita of population on such prevention; dollars spent on such prevention compared to expenditures by the big tobacco companies on advertising, lobbying, and support for political candidates. Nevertheless, a good deal has been accomplished, including effective use of the "stone dropped in the water" approach, that is, use of limited appropriations to create broad coalitions that involve in the effort a wide gamut of nongovernmental organizations: professional; commercial (such as sectors of the pharmaceutical, food, and advertising industries); management and labor; and voluntary, religious, educational, and many other groups.

It is a reasonable inference that this approach, enabling extensive outreach to the population, is importantly related to the progress made. This is despite limited resources and considerable "noise in the system" due to the organized opposition of special commercial interests, including the big tobacco companies, the egg, dairy, and meat industries, as well as the producers of salt and alcoholic beverages. Two of the present-day reprehensible aspects of this opposition is the effort of the tobacco companies to block bans on tobacco advertising in the European community and the United States, and to make up for declining tobacco use in industrialized countries by pushing cigarettes, by every means possible, on the people of the economically developing countries. The undeviating singleness of purpose of these companies was clearly expressed years ago by William Hobbs, president of R.J. Reynolds Tobacco: "If they caused every smoker to smoke just one less cigarette a day, our company would stand to lose $92 million in sales annually. I assure you that we don't intend to let that happen without a fight" [115]. Physicians and other health professionals must, of course, have a different motivation. It is against this background that all of us must be concerned to contend with the fact that as recently as the 1980s in some European countries, the percentage of physicians who still smoked was almost as high as, or even higher than, that of the general population.

Public Response to Efforts for CHD–Stroke–CVD Prevention

Despite the all-too-limited resources allocated for the prevention effort, and the efforts to block it by special interests, the concern of the population, its readiness to respond, and its *positive responses* are documented in data available from several countries. For example, in regard to developments in the United States, with which I am most familiar, they have reached "critical mass" and are of a degree and extent reflected in overall national statistics. These encompass impressive rates of smoking cessation and of decline in the proportion of the population currently smoking and improvements in food intake patterns, including declines in per capita intake of eggs, lard, butter and fat-containing dairy products, beef and other red meats, salt, distilled spirits, and increased intake of skim milk and low-fat milk products, chicken, turkey, fish, fresh fruits, and vegetables [116]. The result has been declines in dietary cholesterol and saturates, with declines in Keys score, and correspondingly, declines in average serum cholesterol of adults, from about 235 mg/dl in the 1950s to 225 in the early 1960s to 205 in the late 1980s–early 1990s [12,19,35,43]. The latest data also indicate that population mean blood pressure levels are down, in part independent of antihypertensive drug treatment. Leisure time exercise has also increased measurably. And the consciousness of the public in regard to these matters finds reflection in a host of ways, ranging from food advertising to cartoon humor. Cholesterol has become a household word!

These are important positive changes. But there are also important shortfalls: Dietary cholesterol intake still averages about 350 mg/day, or about 160 mg/1000 Kcal, above the goal of less than 300 mg/day, or less than 100 mg/1000 Kcal. Dietary saturates are still about 13%–14% of kilocalories, still above the goal of less than 10%. Dietary total fat is about 38% of kilocalories, far above the goal of no more than 30%. And no progress has been registered in the population overall with the problem of epidemic obesity [77,117]. Correspondingly, the adult mean serum cholesterol level of 205 mg/dl is above the national goals set first for 1990, then for the year 2000, of no more than 200 mg/dl [113]. Prevalence rates of frank hypertension remain high, and the majority of the adult population has levels above the optimal of SBP/DBP < 120/< 80 mmHg. About 30% of men and 25% of women still smoke cigarettes.

In regard to these shortfalls, certain trends are of particular concern: recent survey data indicating less favorable dietary practices; adverse patterns among young people; and evidence that throughout these years of progress those of lower socioeconomic status have done much less well than those of higher socioeconomic status [77,117]. This important finding has been registered in several countries.

Trends of CHD–Stroke–CVD–All-Causes Mortality

The "bottom line" is, of course, the trends in regard to the CVD epidemic, and for many countries they have been favorable, dramatically so for some. For example, the pace-setting sustained decline in U.S. CHD mortality rates is about 50% from the peak level of the late 1960s (Fig. 3) [77]. Percentage decline in stroke death rates has been even greater. If the rate of rise in CHD death rates of the 1950s had continued, there would have been about 1 290 000 CHD deaths in 1990 among Americans. If the rates had remained on a plateau at peak levels registered in the late 1960s, there would have been about 980 000 CHD deaths in 1990. There were "only" 491 000. A dramatic reduction indeed. And much evidence is available to support the inference that a considerable proportion of this decline, probably the majority, reflects realization of the potential for prevention, that is, improvements in lifestyles and in the prevention and control of major lifestyle-related risk factors.

As the Japanese experience shows, the Far Eastern pattern of the CVD epidemic, with marked predominance of stroke as the major adult CV disease (rather than CHD), is also amenable to control (Fig. 4) [118]. Remarkable indeed is the long-term trend of decline in stroke mortality in Japan, for both men and women, from highs of over 400/100 000 per year for men and about 300 for women in the 1950s to well under 100 by 1990. And CHD death rates, always much lower than those for stroke, and the lowest of any industrialized country, have declined further.

Obviously, the potential for prevention is realizable on a national and international scale. But to date in every respect—lifestyle improvements, risk-factor decreases, mortality declines—the optimal achievements made by any given country or set of countries are incomplete advances, however impressive. As the 491 000 CHD deaths in the United States in 1990 indicate, the epidemic continues. Its flank has been turned, but it has *not* been ended. And, as several data sets show for several industrialized countries, the downturns in mortality, like the improvements in lifestyles and lifestyle-related risk factors, are much less, or even nonexistent, for those of lower socioeconomic status [77,117]. Moreover, the economically developing countries face a latter-day CHD epidemic.

Clearly then, much needs to be done, both to enhance public policy and its implementation, if the full potential for prevention—the end of the epidemic and its avoidance in the developing countries—is to be realized.

Acknowledgments. It is a pleasure to acknowledge the role of the many individuals and organizations involved in the Chicago Heart Association Detection Project in Industry (CHA) Study, including the 84 cooperating companies; the members of the two survey teams; the staff leadership and responsible committee of the CHA; senior colleagues with executive responsibility for the Project during its years of field work (1967–1973), particularly James A. Schoenberger, MD, and Richard B. Shekelle, PhD; the team accomplishing the serial ascertainment of vital status of the almost 40 000 participants over the years; and colleagues involved in the data editing, analyses, and reporting. The many individuals are listed in several original papers presenting CHA Study results, including reference [5] here. The computer analyses presented here were done by Dan Carside, MA.

It is gratifying also to express appreciation to the officers, executive leadership, and labor force of the Western Electric Company, Chicago, Illinois, USA; their cooperation made the Western Electric (WE) Study possible. It is also a pleasure to acknowledge the role of Oglesby Paul, MD, and Mark Lepper, MD, in the initiation of the WE Study and its leadership for many years; of Ann MacMillan Shryock, BS, in the collection of the nutrition data on the WE men; of the many physicians who participated in the annual examinations of the cohort (see reference [5] for a listing); of Dan Garside and Lois Steinfeldt for maintenance of the WE data files; of Carol Malizia for supervising the 20- and 25-year follow-up surveys; of Ronald Prineas, MD, PhD, and members of the ECG Coding Laboratory, Division of Epidemiology, School of Public Health, University of Minnesota, Minneapolis, Minnesota, USA for ECG coding and quality control.

Appreciation is expressed for the contributions of the many colleagues in the 18 cities in the United States who carried out the Multiple Risk Factor Intervention Trial (MRFIT) and to the group at its Coordinating Center, University of Minnesota, School of Public Health, who have been accomplishing the sequential determination of mortality status of the cohort of 361 662 men screened for MRFIT, and the data editing, processing, and major aspects of the data reporting, particularly James Neaton, PhD, and Deborah Wentworth, who prepared the MRFIT data presented here. Names of the many colleagues and staff in the MRFIT effort over the years are included in its key original reports.

It is gratifying also to acknowledge the contribution of colleagues worldwide to the INTERSALT Study, at the 52 locations in 32 countries where the field work was done; at the Central Laboratory, University of Leuven, Leuven, Belgium; and at the Chicago and London Coordinating Centers (see reference [51] for a listing of individuals). Professor Alan R. Dyer, PhD, did the statistical analyses to produce the coefficients in Table 7 here.

Cooperation is also gratefully acknowledged of the Food and Agriculture Organization (FAO), Rome, Italy, in making available national food balance sheet data and of the World Health Organization (WHO), Geneva, Switzerland in making available age-sex-cause-specific national mortality data. It is also a pleasure to express thanks to Marilyn Buzzard, PhD, Director, and to the staff of the Nutrition Coordinating Center, School of Public Health, University of Minnesota, for the fine work on the nutrient analyses of national food balance sheets from FAO. The data in Fig. 3 are from a chartbook and a report of the National Heart, Lung, and Blood Institute (NHLBI), Bethesda, Maryland, USA; the cooperation of NHLBI is gratefully acknowledged. The INTERSALT data reproduced in Fig. 2 were originally published in the *British Medical Journal*, London, England; the data in Table 3, in *Cardiology*, published by Karger, Basel, Switzerland; the data in Table 7, in the *American Journal of Epidemiology*, Baltimore, Maryland, USA.

The Chicago studies reported here have been supported by the American Heart Association and its Chicago and Illinois affiliates; the National Heart, Lung, and Blood Institute; the Chicago Health Research Foundation; the Otho S. Sprague Foundation; the Research and Education Committee of the Presbyterian-St. Luke's Hospital; the Illini Foundation; and corporate and other private donors. The MRFIT investigation is a collaborative research undertaking with NHLBI contract and grant support. For a listing of the multiple sources of support of the international cooperative INTERSALT Study, see reference [51].

Appreciation is expressed to Professor Rose Stamler for her assistance in the final editing of this paper.

References

1. Stamler J (1981) Primary prevention of epidemic premature atherosclerotic coronary heart disease. In: Yu PM, Goodwin JF (eds) Progress in cardiology, vol 10. Lea and Febiger, Philadelphia, pp 63–100
2. Ruth KJ, Stamler J, Garside D (1993) Trends in dietary fat, cholesterol and coronary heart disease: Ecologic data from 26 countries. Circulation 87:685
3. Stamler J, Garside D, Dyer A, Stamler R, Liu K, Greenland P (1993) The strong positive relationship of serum cholesterol to risk of death from cardiovascular heart disease (CHD), all cardiovascular diseases (CVD), cancers, other diseases and all causes in employed young adult men: Findings of the Chicago Heart Association Study (CHA). Circulation 88[Suppl I]:I-124
4. Mariotti S, Capocaccia R, Farchi G, Menotti A, Verdecchia A, Keys A (1986) Age, period, cohort and geographical area effects on the relationship between risk factors and coronary heart disease mortality: 15-year follow-up of the European cohorts of the Seven Countries Study. J Chron Dis 39:229–242
5. Stamler J, Dyer AR, Shekelle RB, Neaton J, Stamler R (1993) Relationship of baseline major risk factors to coronary and all-cause mortality, and to longevity: Findings from long-term follow-up of Chicago cohorts. Cardiology 82:191–222
6. Klag M, Ford D, Mead L, He J, Whelton PK, Liang K, Levine DM (1993) Serum cholesterol in young men and subsequent cardiovascular disease. N Engl J Med 328:313–318
7. Cornfield J (1962) Joint dependence of risk of coronary heart disease in serum cholesterol and systolic blood pressure: A discriminant function analysis. Fed Proc 21:58–61
8. Stamler J, Wentworth D, Neaton JD (1986) Is relationship between serum cholesterol and risk of premature death from coronary heart disease continuous and graded? Findings in 356,222 primary screenees of the Multiple Risk Factor Intervention Trial (MRFIT). JAMA 256:2823–2828
9. The Lipid Research Clinics Program (1984) The Lipid Research Clinics Coronary Primary Prevention Trial results. I. Reduction in incidence of coronary heart disease. JAMA 251:351–364
10. The Lipid Research Clinics Program (1984) The Lipid Research Clinics Coronary Primary Prevention Trial results. II. The relationship of reduction in incidence of coronary heart disease to cholesterol lowering. JAMA 251:367–374
11. Neaton JD, Blackburn H, Jacobs D, Kuller L, Lee DJ, Sherwin R, Shih J, Stamler J, Wentworth D, for the Multiple Risk Factor Intervention Trial Research Group (1992) Serum cholesterol level and mortality: Findings for the men screened in the Multiple Risk Factor Intervention Trial. Arch Intern Med 152:1490–1500
12. Stamler J, Stamler R, Brown W, Gotto A, Greenland P, Grundy S, Hegsted M, Luepker R, Neaton J, Steinberg D, Stone N, Van Horn L, Wissler R (1993) Serum cholesterol: Doing the right thing. Circulation 88:1954–1960
13. National Center for Health Statistics (1985) United States life tables, United States decennial life tables, vol I/1, DHHS Publication No (PHS) 85-21150-1. United States Government Printing Office, Washington, D.C.

14. The Pathobiological Determinants of Atherosclerosis in Youth (PDAY) Research Group (1990) Relationship of atherosclerosis in young men to serum lipoprotein cholesterol concentrations and smoking. JAMA 264:3018–3024
15. MacMahon S, Peto R, Cutler J, Collins R, Sorlie P, Neaton J, Abbott R, Godwin J, Dyer A, Stamler J (1990) Blood pressure, stroke, and coronary heart disease. Part 1, Prolonged differences in blood pressure: Prospective observational studies corrected for the regression dilution bias. Lancet 335:765–774
16. Keys A (1965) Dietary survey methods in studies on cardiovascular epidemiology. Voeding 26:464–483
17. Liu K, Stamler J, Dyer A, McKeever J, McKeever P (1978) Statistical methods to assess and minimize the role of intra-individual variability in obscuring the relationship between dietary lipids and serum cholesterol. J Chronic Dis 31:399–418
18. Stamler J (1993) Dietary salt and blood pressure. Ann NY Acad Sci 676:122–156
19. Stamler J (1994) Assessing diets to improve world health: Nutritional research on disease causation in populations. Am J Clin Nutr 59:146S–156S
20. Shekelle RB, Shryock AM, Paul O, Lepper M, Stamler J, Liu S, Raynor WJ (1981) Diet, serum cholesterol, and death from coronary heart disease. The Western Electric study. N Engl J Med 304:65–70
21. Burke BS (1947) The dietary history as a tool in research. J Am Diet Assoc 23:1041–1046
22. Shekelle RB, Stamler J (1989) Dietary cholesterol and ischaemic heart disease. Lancet 1:1177–1179
23. Stamler J, Shekelle R (1988) Dietary cholesterol and human coronary heart disease. The epidemiologic evidence. Arch Pathol Lab Med 112:1032–1040
24. Hammond EC (1966) Smoking in relation to the death rates of one million men and women. In: Haenszel W (ed.) Epidemiological Approaches to the Study of Cancer and Other Chronic Diseases. National Cancer Institute Monograph 19. U.S. Department of Health, Education, and Welfare, U.S. Public Health Service, National Cancer Institute, pp 127–204
25. Rose G (1985) Sick individuals and sick populations. Int J Epidemiol 14:32–38
26. Stamler J, Neaton JD, Wentworth D, for the MRFIT Research Group (1994) Mortality of low risk and other men: 16-year follow-up of 353,340 men screened for the Multiple Risk Factor Intervention Trial (MRFIT) (abstract). 34th Annual Conference on Cardiovascular Disease Epidemiology and Prevention, Tampa, Fla., March 16–18, 1994
27. Stamler J, Garside D, Stamler R, Dyer A, Greenland P, Liu D, Ruth KJ (1994) Low risk women and men: 19-year mortality data, Chicago Heart Association Detection Project in Industry (abstract). 34th Annual Conference on Cardiovascular Disease Epidemiology and Prevention, Tampa, Fla., March 16–18, 1994
28. Keys A, Anderson JT, Grande R (1965) Serum cholesterol response to changes in the diet. I. Iodine value of dietary fat versus 2S-P. Metabolism 14:747–758
29. Keys A, Anderson JT, Grande F (1965) Serum cholesterol response to changes in the diet. II. The effect of cholesterol in the diet. Metabolism 14:759–765
30. Keys A, Anderson JT, Grande F (1965) Serum cholesterol response to changes in the diet. III. Differences among individuals. Metabolism 14:766–775
31. Keys A, Anderson JT, Grande F (1965) Serum cholesterol response to changes in the diet. IV. Particular saturated fatty acids in the diet. Metabolism 14:776–787
32. Keys A, Grande F, Anderson JT (1961) Fiber and pectin in the diet and serum cholesterol concentration in man. Proc Soc Exp Biol Med 106:555–562

33. Anderson JT, Lawer A, Keys A (1957) Weight gain from simple overeating. Serum lipids and blood volume. J Clin Invest 36:81–88
34. Hegsted DM, Ausman LM, Johnson JA, Dallal GE (1993) Dietary fat and serum lipids: An evaluation of the experimental data. Am J Clin Nutr 57:875–883
35. Johnson CL, Rifkind BM, Sempos CT, Carroll MD, Bachorik PS, Briefel RR, Gordon DJ, Burt VL, Brown CD, Lippel K, Cleeman JI (1993) Declining serum total cholesterol levels among US adults: The National Health and Nutrition Examination Surveys. JAMA 269:3002–3008
36. National Diet–Heart Study Research Group (1968) The National Diet–Heart Study Final Report. Circulation 37 (Suppl. I):1–428
37. Jenkins DJ, Wolever TM, Rao AV, Hegele RA, Mitchell SJ, Ransom TP, Boctor DL, Spadafora PJ, Jenkins AL, Mehling C (1993) Effect on blood lipids of very high intakes of fiber in diets low in saturated fat and cholesterol. N Engl J Med 329:21–26
38. Lewis B, Hammett F, Katan M, Kay RM, Merkx I, Novels A, Miller NE, Swan AV (1981) Towards an improved lipid-lowering diet: Additive effects of changes in nutrient intake. Lancet 2:1310–1313
39. Van Horn LV, Liu K, Parker D, Emidy L, Liao Y, Pan WH, Giumetti D, Hewitt J, Stamler J (1986) Serum lipid response to oat product intake with a fat-modified diet. J Am Diet Assoc 86:759–764
40. Van Horn L, Emidy LA, Liu KA, Liao YL, Ballew C, King J, Stamler J (1988) Serum lipid response to a fat-modified, oatmeal-enhanced diet. Prev Med 17: 377–386
41. Van Horn L, Moag-Stahlberg A, Liu K, Ballew C, Ruth K, Hughes R, Stamler J (1991) Effects on serum lipids of adding instant oats to usual American diet. Am J Publ Health 81:183–188
42. National Research Council, Committee on Diet and Health, Food and Nutrition Board, Commission on Life Sciences (1989) Diet and health: Implications for reducing chronic disease. Washington, D.C.: National Academy Press
43. Stamler J (1981) Primary prevention of coronary heart disease: The last 20 years. Am J Cardiol 47:722–735
44. Sacks F, Castelli WP, Donner A, Kass EH (1975) Plasma lipids and lipoproteins in vegetarians and controls. N Engl J Med 292:1148–1151
45. Keys A, Aravanis C, Blackburn HW, Van Buchem FS, Buzina R, Djordjevic BD, Dontas AS, Fidanza F, Karvonen MJ, Kimura N, Lekos D, Monti M, Puddu V, Taylor HL (1966) Epidemiological studies related to coronary heart disease: Characteristics of men aged 40–59 in seven countries. Acta Med Scand 460:1–392
46. Keys A (1980) Seven countries—a multivariate analysis of death and coronary heart disease. Harvard University Press, Cambridge, Mass.
47. Stamler R, Stamler J (eds) (1979) Asymptomatic hyperglycemia and coronary heart disease. A series of papers by the International Collaborative Group, based on studies in fifteen populations. J Chronic Dis 32:683–837
48. Stamler J (1979) Population studies. In: Levy RI, Rifkind BM, Dennis BH, Ernst ND (eds) Nutrition, lipids, and coronary heart disease—A global view. Raven Press, New York, pp 25–88
49. People's Republic of China–United States Cardiovascular and Cardiopulmonary Epidemiology Research Group (1992) An epidemiological study of cardiovascular and cardiopulmonary disease risk factors in four populations in the People's

Republic of China: Baseline report from the P.R.C.-U.S.A. Collaborative Study. Circulation 85:1083–1096

50. INTERSALT Cooperative Research Group (authored by Elliott P, Stamler R) (1988) Manual of operations for "INTERSALT"—an international cooperative study on the relation of sodium and potassium to blood pressure. Controlled Clin Trials 9:1S–118S

51. INTERSALT Cooperative Research Group (1988) INTERSALT: An international study of electrolyte excretion and blood pressure. Results for 24 hour urinary sodium and potassium excretion. Br Med J 297:319–328

52. INTERSALT Cooperative Research Group (Elliott P, ed) (1989) The INTERSALT Study—An international cooperative study of electrolyte excretion and blood pressure—further results. J Human Hypertens 3:279–407

53. Elliott P (1989) The INTERSALT study: An addition to the evidence on salt and blood pressure, and some implications. J Human Hypertens 3:289–98

54. Stamler J, Rose G, Stamler R, Elliott P, Dyer A, Marmot M (1989) INTERSALT study findings: Public health and medical care implications. Hypertension 14: 570–577

55. Stamler R (1991) Implications of the INTERSALT Study. Hypertension 17: I-16–I-20

56. Dyer AR, Shipley M, Elliott P for the INTERSALT Cooperative Research Group (1994) Urinary electrolyte excretion in 24 hours and blood pressure in the INTERSALT Study. I. Estimates of reliability. Am J Epidemiol 139:927–939

57. Dyer AR, Shipley M, Elliott P for the INTERSALT Cooperative Research Group (1994) Urinary electrolyte excretion in 24 hours and blood pressure in the INTERSALT Study. II. Estimates of electrolyte-blood pressure associations corrected for regression dilution bias. Am J Epidemiol 139:940–951

58. Joint National Committee on Detection, Evaluation, and Treatment of High Blood Pressure (1993) The fifth report of the Joint National Committee on Detection, Evaluation, and Treatment of High Blood Pressure (JNCV). Arch Intern Med 153:154–183

59. National High Blood Pressure Education Program Working Group (1993) National High Blood Pressure Education Program Working Group report on primary prevention of hypertension. Arch Intern Med 153:186–208

60. Cutler JA, Kotchen TA, Obarzanek E (eds) (1991) The National Heart, Lung, and Blood Institute Workshop on Salt and Blood Pressure. Hypertension 17[Suppl I]:I-1–I-221

61. Stamler R, Stamler J, Grimm R, Gosch FC, Elmer P, Dyer A, Berman R, Fishman J, Van Heel N, Civinelli J, McDonald A (1987) Nutritional therapy for high blood pressure. Final report of a four-year randomized controlled trial—the Hypertension Control Program. JAMA 257:1484–1491

62. Stamler R, Stamler J, Gosch FC, Civinelli J, Fishman J, McKeever P, McDonald A, Dyer AR (1989) Primary prevention of hypertension by nutritional-hygienic means. Final report of a randomized, controlled trial. JAMA 262:1801–1807

63. Law MR, Frost CD, Wald NJ (1991) By how much does salt restriction lower blood pressure? I. Analysis of observational data among populations. II. Analysis of observational data within populations. III. Analysis of data from trials of salt reduction. Br Med J 302:811–824

64. Forte JG, Miguel JM, Miguel MJ, De Padua F, Rose G (1989) Salt and blood pressure: A community trial. J Human Hypertens 3:179–184

65. Stamler R, Shipley M, Elliott P, Dyer A, Sans S, Stamler J, on behalf of the INTERSALT Cooperative Research Group (1992) Higher blood pressure in adults with less education: Some likely explanatory factors. Findings of the INTERSALT Study. Hypertension 19:237–241

66. Elliott P, Kesteloot H, Dyer A, Freeman J, Shipley M, Stamler J, Rose G, Marmot M, Stamler R (1992) 24-hour urinary nitrogen excretion and blood pressure: INTERSALT findings. Circulation 84:II-698

67. Dyer A, Elliott P, Kesteloot H, Stamler J, Stamler R, Freeman J, Shipley M, Marmot M, Rose G (1992) Urinary nitrogen excretion and blood pressure in INTERSALT. J Hypertens 10:S122

68. Kihara M, Fujikawa J, Ohtaka M, Mano M, Nara Y, Horie R, Tsunematsu T, Note S, Fukase M, Yamori Y (1984) Interrelationships between blood pressure, sodium, potassium, serum cholesterol, and protein intake in Japanese. Hypertension 6: 736–742

69. Yamori Y, Kigara M, Nara Y, Ohtaka M, Horie R, Tsunematsu T, Note S, Fukase M (1981) Hypertension and diet: Multiple regression analysis in a Japanese farming community. Lancet 1:1204–1205

70. Zhou Bei-fang, Wu Xi-gui, Tao Shou-qi, et al (1988) Dietary patterns in 10 groups and their relationship with blood pressure. Chin Med J 102:257–261

71. Shang X, Cai R, Zhou B (1993) The relationships of dietary protein, serum and urine free amino acids and blood pressure in three Chinese populations (abstract). 3rd International Conference on Preventive Cardiology, Oslo, Norway, 27 June–1 July 1993

72. Stamler J, Caggiula A, Grandits GA (1992) Habitual intake of minerals, fiber, alcohol, caffeine, macronutrients and systolic blood pressure (SBP): 6-year data on 12000+ MRFIT men. J Hypertens 10:S143

73. Liu K, Ruth KJ, Shekelle RB, Stamler J (1993) Macronutrients and long-term change in systolic blood pressure. Circulation 87:2

74. Liu K, Ruth K, Flack J, Burke G, Savage P, Liang KY, Hardin M, Hulley S (1992) Ethnic differences in 5-year blood pressure change in young adults: The CARDIA Study. Circulation 85:867

75. Elliott P, Freeman J, Pryer J, Brenner E, Marmot M (1992) Dietary protein and blood pressure: A report from the dietary and nutritional survey of British adults. J Hypertens 10:S141

76. Stamler J, Ruth KJ, Liu K, Shekelle RB (1994) Dietary antioxidents and blood pressure change in the Western Electric Study, 1958–1966 (abstract). 34th Annual Conference on Cardiovascular Disease Epidemiology and Prevention, Tampa, Fla., March 16–18, 1994

77. Oberman A, Kuller LH, Carleton RA, Blackburn J, Stamler J, et al (1994) National Heart, Lung, and Blood Institute Report of the Task Force on Epidemiology and Prevention of Cardiovascular Diseases. U.S. Department of Health and Human Services, Public Health Service, National Institute of Health, pp i–xv and 1–130

78. Multiple Risk Factor Intervention Trial Research Group (1990) Mortality rates after 10.5 years for participants in the Multiple Risk Factor Intervention Trial— Findings related to a prior hypothesis of the trial. JAMA 263:1795–1801

79. World Health Organization European Collaborative Group (1986) European collaborative trial of multifactorial prevention of coronary heart disease: Final report on the 6-year results. Lancet 1:869–872

80. Rose G (1987) European collaborative trial of multifactorial prevention of coronary heart disease. Lancet 1:685
81. Holme I, Hjerrmann I, Helgeland A, Leren P (1985) The Oslo Study: Diet and anti-smoking advice. Additional results from a five-year primary preventive trial in middle-age men. Prev Med 14:279–292
82. Hjermann I (1993) Non-pharmacological prevention of coronary heart disease. Presented at 61st meeting, European Atherosclerosis Society, Capri, Italy, May 18, 1993
83. Wilhelmsen L, Berglund G, Elmfeldt D, Tibblin G, Wedel H, Pennert K, Vedin A, Wilhelmsen C, Werko L (1986) The multifactor primary prevention trial in Goteborg, Sweden. Eur Heart J 7:279–288
84. Page IH, Allen EV, Chamberlain FL, Keys A, Stamler J, Stare FJ (1961) Dietary fat and its relation to heart attacks and strokes. Circulation 23:133–136
85. Inter-Society Commission for Heart Disease Resources (1970) Atherosclerosis Study Group and Epidemiology Study Group. Primary Prevention of the Atherosclerotic Diseases. Circulation 42:A55–A95
86. Grundy SM, Bilheimer D, Blackburn H, Brown V, Kwiterovich P, Mattson F, Schonfeld G, Weidman W (1982) Rationale of the diet-heart statement of the American Heart Association. Report of Nutrition Committee. Circulation 65: 839A-854A
87. Keys A (1968) Official collective recommendations on diet in the Scandinavian countries. Nutr Rev 26:259–263
88. WHO Expert Committee on the Prevention of Coronary Heart Disease (1982) Expert Committee Report on the prevention of coronary heart disease. World Health Organization, Technical Report Series No 678, Geneva, Switzerland
89. Muldoon MF, Manuck SB, Matthews KA (1990) Lowering cholesterol concentrations and mortality: A quantitative review of primary prevention trials. Br Med J 301:309–314
90. Ravnskov U (1992) Cholesterol lowering trials in coronary heart disease: Frequency of citation and outcome. Br Med J 305:15–19
91. Schmidt JG (1992) Cholesterol lowering treatment and mortality. Br Med J 305:1226–1227
92. The Coronary Drug Project Research Group (1970) The Coronary Drug Project: Initial findings leading to modifications of its research protocol. JAMA 214: 1303–1313
93. The Coronary Drug Project Research Group (1972) The Coronary Drug Project: Findings leading to further modifications of its protocol with respect to dextrothyroxine. JAMA 220:996–1008
94. Coronary Drug Project Research Group (1973) The Coronary Drug Project: Findings leading to discontinuation of the 2.5 mg/day estrogen group. JAMA 226:652–657
95. Coronary Drug Project Research Group (1983) The Coronary Drug Project: Methods and lessons of a multicenter clinical trial. Controlled Clin Trials 4: 273–541
96. Coronary Drug Project Research Group (1975) The Coronary Drug Project: Clofibrate and niacin in coronary heart disease. JAMA 231:360–381
97. Canner PL, Berge KG, Wenger NK, Stamler J, Friedman L, Prineas RJ, Friedewald W (1986) Fifteen year mortality in Coronary Drug Project patients: Long-term benefit with niacin. J Am Coll Cardiol 8:1245–1255

98. Kleinman LC (1992) To end an epidemic. Lessons from the history of diphtheria. N Engl J Med 326:773–777
99. Kleinman LC (1993) Control of epidemics (letter to editor). N Engl J Med 328:667
100. Mann JM (1993) AIDS in the 1990's: A global analysis. Pharos 56:2–5
101. White PD, Sprague HB, Stamler J, Stare FJ, Wright IS, Katz LN, Levine SL, Page IH (1959) A statement on arteriosclerosis, main cause of "heart attacks" and "strokes". National Health Education Council, New York
102. American Heart Association Committee Report (1980) Risk factors and coronary disease—a statement for physicians. Circulation 62:449A-455A
103. Chait A, Brunzell JD, Denke MA, Eisenberg K, Ernst ND, Franklin FA, Ginsberg H, Kotchen TA, Kuller L, Mullis RM, Nichaman MZ, Nicolosi RJ, Schaefer EJ, Stone NJ, Weidman WH (1993) Rationale of the Diet-Heart Statement of the American Heart Association. Report of the Nutrition Committee. Circulation 88:3008–3029
104. Advisory Committee to the Surgeon General (1964) Smoking and Health. U.S. Department of Health, Education and Welfare, Washington, D.C.
105. U.S. Department of Agriculture/Department of Health and Human Services (1990) Nutrition and your health: Dietary guidelines for Americans, 3rd edn. U.S. Goverment Printing Office, Home and Garden Bulletin No 232, Washington, D.C.
106. U.S. Department of Health and Human Services (1988) The Surgeon General's Report on Nutrition and Health. U.S. Government Printing Office, Washington, D.C.
107. National Cholesterol Education Program (1990) Report of the Expert Panel on population strategies for blood cholesterol reduction. U.S. Department of Health and Human Services, Public Health Services, National Institutes of Health Publication No 90-3046
108. National Cholesterol Education Program (1991) Report of the Expert Panel on blood cholesterol levels in children and adolescents. U.S. Department of Health and Human Services, Public Health Services, National Institutes of Health Publication No 91-2732
109. Expert Panel On Detection, Evaluation, and Treatment of High Blood Cholesterol In Adults (1993) Summary of the Second Report of the National Cholesterol Education Program (NCEP) Expert Panel on Detection, Evaluation, and Treatment of High Blood Cholesterol in Adults (Adult Treatment Panel II). JAMA 269:3015–3023
110. U.S. Department of Health, Education, and Welfare (1990) Smoking and health: A report of the Surgeon General. U.S. Government Printing Office, Washington, D.C.
111. U.S. Department of Health, Education, and Welfare (1991) Smoking and health: A report of the Surgeon General. U.S. Government Printing Office, Washington, D.C.
112. U.S. Department of Health, Education, and Welfare (1992) Smoking and health: A report of the Surgeon General. U.S. Government Printing Office, Washington, D.C.
113. U.S. Department of Health and Human Services (1991) Healthy People 2000: National health promotion and disease prevention objectives (summary report). DHHS Publication No (PHS) 91–50213. Public Health Service; U.S. Government Printing Office, Washington, D.C.

114. Rose G (1992) The strategy of preventive medicine. Oxford University Press, New York
115. Chapman S, Woodward S (1991) Australian court rules that passive smoking causes lung cancer, asthma attacks, and respiratory disease. Br Med J 302:943–945
116. U.S. Bureau of the Census (1992) Statistical abstract of the United States: 1992, 112th edn. U.S. Government Printing Office, Washington, D.C.
117. Stamler J (1993) Epidemic obesity in the United States. Arch Intern Med 153: 1040–1044
118. Data from the World Health Organization, Geneva

Discussion

Asian-Pacific student: Would you comment on using low birth weight in the prediction of coronary heart disease in adults, a big controversy in my country?

J. Stamler: An interesting development in cardiovascular disease epidemiology has been the research of David Barker, a colleague of Geoffrey Rose, on the ecological and individual associations between nutritional deprivation of the fetus and infant and possible long-term effects on adult diseases. Risk of diabetes, of hypertension, and hypercholesterolemia may very well be part of socioeconomic phenomena, reflecting problems from conception on. There are important confounders in those studies, but it is a fascinating new area of research. It contradicts nothing that we have learned about adults, but underscores the importance of problems not only from the cradle but from conception to the grave.

R. Bonita: You have made wonderful progress in North America in improving lifestyle. Can you comment on the concern that some of us have about the trade agreements that America is imposing, particularly in regard to tobacco?

J. Stamler: I don't have enough information about our trade agreements to make intelligent comments on them. However, it is clear that official U.S. "pushing" of American tobacco products on developing countries is bad policy.

Asian-Pacific Seminar student: A. I have heard a great deal this week about changing risk factors and habits in adults but nothing about such changes in children. Would you comment?

J. Stamler: It is an inevitable consequence of everything that has emerged in this field that the key is prevention of risk factors themselves. Clearly adults need help, but it is late, it is defensive, it is endless, because it doesn't address the basic problem, that is, control and elimination of risk factor early, *long before* problems develop. This involves social policy as well as medical care and includes the homes, and schools, the food supply, and all the broad social determinants of health.

To me it has always been sensible and possible through effective public health policy to influence parents' and youths' eating patterns to achieve average teenage and young adult cholesterol levels around 150–160 mg/dl, and no further rise with age, as was true in Japan. There are cultures in which blood pressure as well does not increase with age from youth on. Thus, preventing rise in blood pressure is possible, and the time to begin is early in childhood, with the primary creation of healthy habits of eating, exercising, of not smoking, of using alcohol sensibly. That may seem difficult at the moment. But it is necessary and possible.

When we began all this in the 1950s–1960s, if we had said that the coronary death rate is going to be down 50% and the stroke rate down 60% in 30 years, we would have been called crazy. Based on that experience, the possibility exists of achieving improved nutrition through health promotion and appropriate control of the influence of some commercial interests that have money-making, not public health, on their agenda. The cigarette and salt industry are not learning this point, though other industries are. When you see CVD death rates 1/10 that of the rest of the population, among people with low levels of combined risk factors, even in the US, you can project this to the goal of epidemic disease not existing.

Asian-Pacific Seminar student: Indonesia has had two "invasions." One is Marlboro cigarettes, and the second is sodium glutamate. It is difficult for the medical profession to fight against these commercial powers.

J. Stamler: We cannot spell out for other countries how they should do what they need to do. But at an international level, there are some important things that we can talk about. The ISFC voted in Oslo to organize an effective national and international campaign to reduce and eventually end smoking among physicians.

Second, those of us in Britain and the US, where dwell the big tobacco companies who are attempting to make up for declining sales by increasing sales in developing countries, must fight them, including the politicians who put pressure on countries to buy British and American tobacco products in order to maintain favored-nation trading status. Even a former Prime Minister of Britain, for a large sum of money, has become an instrument for international tobacco-promoting sales in the developing world. We must get the international cigarette cartel off the back of developing countries!

For your country's effort, you have to find your own way, consulting with experienced people, and not underestimating the power of organized groups. A main lesson from the US is that it *is* possible to organize public policy through voluntary bodies such as heart foundations.

R. Buzina: The international community cannot go very far intervening into particular governmental policy. But at the WHO-FAO meeting recently in Rome, 160 ministers of health and agriculture signed a declaration for the prevention of chronic diseases, including a strong statement on smoking, signed also by the Minister of Health of Japan. This declaration can be obtained from WHO in Geneva, and provides a good basis for initiating action.

Closing Remarks

HENRY BLACKBURN

You have all been very perseverant. Please persevere two minutes longer! I first want to acknowledge the people who brought us together, Drs. Toshima and Koga and colleagues:

Friends, we have been amazed at your hospitality and at your vision in arranging this milestone conference. May I call on the Seven Countries investigators, joined by all of us here, to express appreciation to Dr. Toshima and his colleague Dr. Koga for putting on this splendid conference. Thank you.

(Applause)

The proceedings of this conference will be published. All attending will receive notification of how to order the publication. In addition to these scientific proceedings, there will be published a personalized history of the Seven Countries adventure that we have had together, composed by the principal investigators themselves and published through Kromhout's enterprise by the Dutch Heart Foundation, with other support from Japan and from Minnesota. You will all be notified of the publisher and cost through Dr. Kromhout's office and the International Edition of the CVD Epidemiology Newsletter.

At this time I would like for all the senior Seven Countries investigators, and their spouses, followed by all study staff, to come to the front of the room for acknowledgement. Thank you!

(Applause)

Will Madame Chika Kimura and Dr. and Mrs. Keys come front to be joined by our guest speakers and intellectual companions along the way: Fred Epstein and Jeremiah Stamler. Thank you, all!

In closing, I hope that all who participated in this historic meeting have come to feel the intellectual excitement of this scientific undertaking, and are impressed with the new generation of investigators, their vigor and vision of the future. I hope that all present will now feel closely involved intellectually with the Seven Countries Study. Thank you.

Professor H. Toshima then closed the ceremonies.

Index